CNOR®

Exam

Practice Questions

CNOR® Practice Tests & Review for the
CNOR® Exam

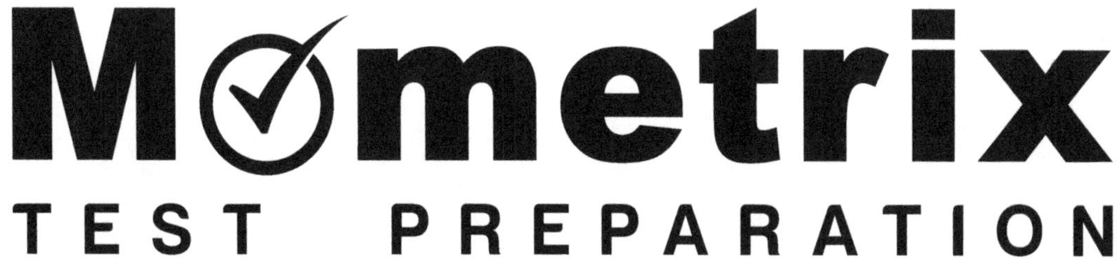

Written and edited the Mometrix Nursing Certification Test Team

Mometrix offers volume discount pricing to institutions. For more information or a price quote, please contact our sales department at sales@mometrix.com or 888-248-1219.

Paperback
ISBN 13: 978-1-62120-044-4
ISBN 10: 1-62120-044-2

Ebook
ISBN 13: 978-1-62120-518-0
ISBN 10: 1-62120-518-5

Hardback
ISBN 13: 978-1-5167-0795-9
ISBN 10: 1-5167-0795-8

DEAR FUTURE EXAM SUCCESS STORY

First of all, **THANK YOU** for purchasing Mometrix study materials!

Second, congratulations! You are one of the few determined test-takers who are committed to doing whatever it takes to excel on your exam. **You have come to the right place.** We developed these practice tests with one goal in mind: to deliver you the best possible approximation of the questions you will see on test day.

Standardized testing is one of the biggest obstacles on your road to success, which only increases the importance of doing well in the high-pressure, high-stakes environment of test day. Your results on this test could have a significant impact on your future, and these practice tests will give you the repetitions you need to build your familiarity and confidence with the test content and format to help you achieve your full potential on test day.

Your success is our success

We would love to hear from you! If you would like to share the story of your exam success or if you have any questions or comments in regard to our products, please contact us at **800-673-8175** or **support@mometrix.com**.

Thanks again for your business and we wish you continued success!

Sincerely,
The Mometrix Test Preparation Team

Written and edited by the Mometrix Exam Secrets Test Prep Team
Printed in the United States of America

TABLE OF CONTENTS

CNOR Practice Test #1

1. The best methods to identify the preoperative patient at a first encounter, before beginning the assessment, is to

a. compare his wristband and chart, and ask him to spell his name.
b. call his name and if he responds, compare his chart and wristband.
c. check his chart, ask the patient to spell his name, and ask the Holding Area nurse to identify him.
d. confirm the patient's identity with his relatives, check his wristband, and ask the Holding Area nurse to identify him.

2. Proper use of the table strap includes

a. applying the table strap after the patient is asleep.
b. positioning the table strap 2 inches above the patient's knees.
c. positioning the table strap 2 inches below the patient's knees.
d. removing the table strap as soon as the patient is extubated.

3. The OR surfaces that require the most attention from cleaners are

a. vertical surfaces.
b. horizontal surfaces.
c. metal surfaces.
d. glass surfaces.

4. The best response when a scrub nurse drops a sterile, single-use item on the floor and does not have a replacement for it is to

a. flash sterilize it.
b. send it to CSS for reprocessing.
c. soak it in alkaline glutaraldehyde for 20 minutes.
d. cancel the case.

5. The circulating nurse stands by the patient during induction in order to do all of the following EXCEPT

a. offer emotional support to the patient.
b. prevent patient falls.
c. observe the sterile set-up.
d. assist the anesthetist.

6. The danger posed when the nurse positions the overhead lights for the upcoming surgery prior to bringing the patient into the Operating Room is

a. head injuries.
b. fires.
c. contamination.
d. enhanced anxiety for the patient.

7. The equipment a perioperative nurse must prepare for an orthopedic case with a Bier Block are

a. two tourniquets or one double-cuffed tourniquet, an Esmarch bandage, and a local anesthetic.
b. a spinal tray, extra pillows, a leg holder, an Esmarch bandage, and a local anesthetic.
c. an epidural catheter, a local anesthetic, and prep solution.
d. xylocaine, a 20 mL syringe, prep solution, a blood pressure monitor, and a pulse oximeter.

8. The best response when a pointed towel clip has penetrated a drape comes unclasped (but remains in place) is to

a. remove the towel clip and replace it with another one.
b. if the towel clip is visible, re-clasp it.
c. ignore the towel clip.
d. ask the circulating nurse to remove the towel clip.

9. One safety measure used in the OR to prevent fires is to

a. never use less than 100% oxygen during facial surgery.
b. shave all beards and mustaches prior to facial surgery.
c. remove unnecessary foot pedals from around surgeon's feet.
d. keep the electrosurgery pencil on the field, so the surgeon can reach it easily.

10. A perioperative nurse prepares for a scheduled surgery by opening the sterile packs and instruments. The scrub nurse sets up. The float nurse informs her there will be a two-hour delay. Her best response is

a. cover the sterile tables before she and the scrub nurse go to lunch.
b. take turns with the scrub nurse to constantly monitor the sterile fields.
c. discard the sterile set-up and order a new one from CSS.
d. leave the OR doors open, so the float nurse can check the sterile fields when passing, and offer to help in another room.

11. Usually, the first medication given for anaphylaxis is

a. epinephrine.
b. albuterol.
c. corticosteroids.
d. antihistamines (H_1 and H_2 blocker).

12. The correct reaction for the circulating nurse who finds the sponge count is incorrect following an open abdominal procedure is to

a. inform the surgeon and anesthesiologist; call Radiology for an abdominal x-ray.
b. inform the surgeon; send the patient to the Post Anesthesia Care Unit (PACU); and continue to search for the sponge.
c. send the patient to the PACU; continue to search for the sponge; if it is not found, file an Incident Report.
d. call the supervisor; send the patient to the PACU; continue to search; if the sponge is not found, inform patient's family.

13. The cleanser that the AORN recommends for showering a preoperative patient is

a. Dove soap.
b. povidone iodine.
c. chlorhexidine gluconate (CHG).
d. alcohol.

14. During x-ray studies of the hips and femur, lead shielding should be applied

a. to protect the thyroid.
b. to protect the ovaries or testes.
c. to protect the other leg.
d. no shielding is necessary.

15. The LEAST likely effect to the OR from a high school class observing a case with the patient's permission is

a. improved public relations and increased interest in surgical careers.
b. increased microorganism colonies.
c. increased risk of surgical site infection (SSI).
d. increased traffic and changes in traffic patterns.

16. The most common cause of toxic anterior segment syndrome (TASS) is

a. contamination with powder from surgical gloves.
b. improper cleaning and sterilization of instruments.
c. improper positioning during surgery.
d. leakage of anesthetic gases.

17. The best response when a preoperative patient tells the perioperative nurse that he developed a high fever during his last surgical procedure is to

a. explain to the patient that his elevated temperature was more than likely due to an infection, and that if it recurs during this procedure, the anesthesiologist will administer antibiotics.
b. page the anesthesiologist and the surgeon; ask them if they want to order a muscle biopsy and precautions for malignant hyperthermia.
c. comfort the patient by telling him the OR is cooled by air conditioning set on "low", and the anesthesiologist will monitor his body temperature at all times.
d. explain that his body temperature may have risen as a response to the cool OR, and then give the patient a warm blanket.

18. An important consideration for scheduling cases in the OR include all of the following EXCEPT

a. staffing availability.
b. specialty room availability (e.g., for an open-heart case).
c. staff lunch schedule.
d. patient background (infectious diseases, length of case).

19. The scrub nurse discards soiled sponges into the kick-buckets. The acceptable technique for the circulating nurse to handle and count soiled sponges is

a. donning gloves and/or utilizing a sponge stick, the circulator places sponges in a pocketed count bag, generally containing 10 visible pockets, one for each sponge. The sponges are then counted throughout the surgery and during the final count before closure.
b. the circulator wears gloves, or uses a sponge stick to handle all sponges. The circulator counts sponges with the scrub nurse or technician. When 5 or 10 accumulate, the circulator places them in a plastic bag and ties it closed, documenting the count in each closed bag.
c. the circulator lines up all soiled sponges across an impervious pad on the floor, so all sponges are clearly visible for the final count. The count is performed after the procedure is complete, then the sponges are discarded in a plastic bag.
d. the circulator wears gloves or uses a sponge stick to place all soiled sponges in bags of 5 or 10. The circulator only performs the final count with scrub nurse.

20. The best fire extinguisher for OR use is

a. carbon dioxide.
b. halon.
c. pressurized water.
d. sodium bicarbonate.

21. Which of the following may cause injury during facial surgery?

a. Avoiding the use of 100% oxygen (O_2) to prevent fire.
b. Draping the patient to prevent pockets of oxygen (O_2) from accumulating.
c. Trimming the patient's facial hair to minimize flammability.
d. Coating the patient's facial hair with a water-soluble lubricant.

22. When assisting a patient with deep-breathing and coughing exercises following major abdominal surgery, the nurse notes that the patient has diminished cough and reduced right basilar breath sounds. The patient reports feeling slightly short of breath and has a low-grade fever. These signs and symptoms are most likely the result of

a. pneumonia.
b. atelectasis.
c. pulmonary edema.
d. pulmonary embolism.

23. Which of the following statements is true regarding an Army-Navy retractor?

a. An Army-Navy retractor is self-retaining.
b. An Army-Navy retractor is like a Balfour with a blade.
c. An Army-Navy retractor is double-ended.
d. An Army-Navy retractor contains a suction port.

24. The surgical team is preparing to turn an intubated surgical patient from supine to prone. One safety technique that must be used when turning a patient into this position is to

a. move quickly to minimize stress on the patient's joints and decrease risk of complications mid-turn.
b. move slowly to ensure the prone position is reached smoothly and gently.
c. delegate one person to the head, and a second to the trunk, to turn the patient.
d. roll the patient by pulling at the patient's arm and hip simultaneously.

25. The appropriate technique for the circulating nurse to remove a contaminated glove from a member of the surgical team is to

a. pull the gown cuff down over the co-worker's hand.
b. do not pull down the gown cuff.
c. grasp the contaminated glove close to the co-worker's wrist, remove it inside out, and discard it.
d. A and C.

26. All of the following are recommended measures to reduce perioperative noise EXCEPT

a. lower ringtone volumes.
b. place pagers and cell phones on silent/vibration mode.
c. use overhead pages instead of text messaging.
d. reduce the number of people present to essential staff.

27. The synonym meaning "suprapubic incision" is

a. midabdominal transverse incision.
b. subcostal incision.
c. Pfannenstiel incision.
d. lower oblique inguinal incision.

28. The best precaution before wrapping an Esmarch bandage around a patient's arm is to

a. lower the arm to allow for venous stasis.
b. raise the arm to allow for venous drainage.
c. scrub the arm with povidone prep solution (Betadine).
d. shave and then scrub the arm with povidone prep solution (Betadine).

29. A patient with a nursing diagnosis of activity intolerance following a total hip arthroplasty has been resistive to mobilization efforts, noting that her friend fell after a hip replacement and dislocated the hip, causing severe pain. The most likely cause of the patient's activity intolerance is

a. physical.
b. motivational.
c. psychological.
d. environmental.

30. All of the following can result from over pressurization during abdominal insufflation with CO_2 EXCEPT

a. hypocarbia.
b. postoperative neck and shoulder pain.
c. decreased respiratory effort and cardiac output.
d. regurgitation and aspiration.

31. Before anesthesia induction, the minimum prewarming time to reduce the risk of hypothermia is:

a. 5 minutes
b. 10 minutes
c. 20 minutes
d. 30 minutes

32. Which of the following essential information required for the perioperative nurse assessment is performed in the Holding Area?

a. Patient's exact age and weight.
b. Allergies, metal implants, and pacemakers.
c. Type and exact location of the surgery.
d. B and C.

33. The method the perioperative nurse uses to alleviate patient anxiety and fear preoperatively is

a. attentive listening and reassurance.
b. promising the patient that everything will be ok.
c. telling the patient that there is nothing to fear.
d. speaking to the patient as a method of distracting them from the process and preparation.

34. All of the following are true about draping a patient for an abdominal incision EXCEPT

a. discard a contaminated drape.
b. avoid shaking or fanning drapes.
c. adjust position of the drape if incorrectly placed.
d. hold drapes above the level of the waist until properly placed.

35. The emphasis of the *Perioperative Patient Focused Model* is on

a. the outcome-driven nature of perioperative patient care.
b. implementation of the care plan.
c. prevention of injury.
d. elimination of risk.

36. All of the following nonverbal communications are common signs of anxiety EXCEPT

a. making eye contact.
b. licking lips, scratching.
c. tapping of the foot.
d. rubbing hands together.

37. What is a *suture memory* and how is it eliminated?

a. *Suture memory* means the suture material returns to its original configuration; gently stretch it without applying tension to its swaged section.
b. *Suture memory* refers to a suture material made from metal; bend it until it is straight.
c. *Suture memory* refers to a suture that knots easily; dip it in water prior to passing it to the surgeon.
d. *Suture memory* refers to a suture that has to be loaded onto a needle; load several needle holders at once.

38. The members of the perioperative health care team responsible for identifying performance improvement projects are

a. administrative staff.
b. perioperative nurses.
c. surgeons.
d. all staff.

39. Which of the following medications is contraindicated for treatment of malignant hyperthermia?

a. Dantrolene sodium.
b. Regular insulin in 50% glucose solution.
c. Calcium chloride.
d. Calcium channel blocker.

40. After it is untied by the perioperative nurse, the soiled gown worn during surgery is removed by first grasping and pulling

a. one sleeve.
b. the neck of the gown.
c. one shoulder seam.
d. one side seam.

41. The proper testing technique to determine if effective sterilization occurred is a

a. biological indicator containing known, living, highly resistant spores.
b. chemical indicator, which changes in color.
c. thermal indicator, which changes in color.
d. bacterial vial with live bacteria.

42. The safety precaution the scrub nurse takes when preparing for invasive surgery is to

a. double-glove.
b. wear an x-ray apron under the sterile gown.
c. wear high booties over shoes.
d. wear a laser high-filtration mask.

43. The heat-generating equipment that must not contact the patient's drape, in case its connectors detach, is/are the

a. fiber-optic cords.
b. electrosurgery cords.
c. suction tubing.
d. laser cords.

44. The agent least likely to be responsible for anaphylaxis during surgery is

a. Isosulfan blue 1%.
b. anesthetic agents (e.g., halothane, isoflurane).
c. latex.
d. antibiotics (penicillin, cephalosporins, sulfonamides).

45. Using the SBAR communication process with a physician, situation ("S") should include

a. a brief statement of problem.
b. the admitting diagnosis.
c. current vital signs.
d. a request for orders.

46. Intravasation of fluids during surgery may result in clinically significant

a. hyponatremia.
b. hypernatremia.
c. hyperkalemia.
d. hypomagnesemia.

47. During the turnover between patients, floor cleaning with an EPA-approved disinfectant should include

a. the entire OR floor.
b. only visibly soiled areas of the floor (such as from blood).
c. 5- to 6-foot perimeter around operating table and visibly spoiled areas.
d. 3- to 4-foot perimeter around operating table and visibly soiled areas.

48. The most common complications the patient may sustain during extubation include all of the following EXCEPT

a. vomiting (emesis).
b. laryngospasm.
c. hyperventilation.
d. bronchospasm.

49. The iatrogenic diseases caused by exposure to anesthetic gases include all of the following EXCEPT

a. leukemia and heart disease.
b. miscarriages and reduced fertility.
c. liver and renal diseases.
d. neurological diseases.

50. The TRUE statement regarding a Jackson Pratt (JP) and a Hemovac drain is

a. JP and Hemovac are the only closed systems that minimize bacteria entering the wound, and permit accurate drainage measurement.
b. they are simple-lumened drains that lie flat under the dressing.
c. they are double-lumened drains that can be attached to external suction.
d. a JP drains a surgical site of small amounts of fluid and blood, whereas the larger Hemovac is both a drain and a device for autologous retransfusion.

51. The nurse is developing a plan of care for a woman who speaks Spanish and minimal English, but brought her 10-year-old daughter to translate. The nurse should

a. call for an adult medical translator.
b. simplify language so the daughter can translate more easily.
c. use pictures and signs and simple language to communicate with the woman.
d. ask the housekeeper, who speaks Spanish, to translate.

52. Risk factors for malignant hyperthermia include all of the following EXCEPT

a. age younger than 15.
b. family history of sudden death after surgery.
c. thin physique with underdeveloped muscles.
d. Duchenne muscular dystrophy.

53. All of the following are precautions that the perioperative nurse takes to avoid plume formation (smoke) during electrosurgery EXCEPT

a. suction with an in-line filter to evacuate smoke.
b. leave OR doors open to vent smoke into the hallway.
c. wear a laser mask to avoid inhaling the smoke plume.
d. have a free-standing smoke evacuator in the case of large amounts of smoke.

54. The correct order for the scrub nurse's sponge count is

a. first count the sponges on the Mayo stand, then the sponges on the surgical field.
b. first count the sponges nearest the patient's incision, secondly the sponges on sticks, thirdly sponges on the Mayo stand, and finally the sponges on the back table.
c. first count unopened packs on the back table, secondly sponges on the Mayo stand, and finally the surgical field, including sponge sticks.
d. first count the circulating nurse's soiled sponges, secondly the surgical field and sponge sticks, thirdly the Mayo stand, and finally the back table.

55. A close personal friend of the perioperative nurse requires an admission assessment and evaluation. The best procedure is

a. complete the assessment unless the patient objects.
b. ask the patient if she would like a different nurse.
c. arrange for a different nurse to complete the assessment.
d. complete the assessment, documenting the relationship on the patient record.

56. A perioperative nurse wears a sterile gown and gloves. The surgeon asks him to come to the opposite side of the OR table. The most appropriate way to pass by other gowned and gloved staff is

a. front-to-front.
b. with his back to the operating table, and his front to the other staffer.
c. back-to-back.
d. side-to-side.

57. The scrub nurse requests more lap sponges from the circulating nurse, who is on a major case. Since the circulating nurse is phoning Pathology, he quickly passes the sponges, but allows the scrub nurse to count them while he relays the report to the surgeon. The TRUE statement regarding this action is

a. the circulating nurse should first relay the Pathology report to the surgeon, then count with the scrub nurse.
b. the circulating nurse should quickly count with the scrub nurse, and then relay the Pathology report to the surgeon.
c. the scrub nurse may count the sponges alone, providing she speaks loudly.
d. the circulating nurse must count the sponges, then pass that report to the scrub nurse.

58. The surgical team's signs and symptoms when there is exhaled anesthetic gas in the OR include all of the following EXCEPT

a. dizziness and nausea.
b. fatigue, drowsiness, and decreased mental acuity.
c. hyperactivity, diaphoresis, and decreased body temperature.
d. headaches.

59. While prepping a patient for electrosurgery, the perioperative nurse notices the dispersive electrode pad is a different brand than the cautery machine. The most appropriate action is to

a. call Central Sterilizing or check the supply room for a matching dispersive pad.
b. use the current pad; they are all interchangeable.
c. inform the surgeon and give him a hand-held cautery device that does not require a dispersive electrode.
d. place the dispersive electrode pad on the patient, without attaching it to the generator.

60. Prophylactic antibiotics should be administered

a. 30 minutes to 1 hour preoperatively.
b. 4-8 hours preoperatively.
c. 12 hours preoperatively.
d. 24 hours preoperatively.

61. Cardiac output is a function of the patient's heart rate and which other factor?

a. Pedal pulse.
b. Stroke volume.
c. Respiratory rate.
d. Glasgow coma scale.

62. The TRUE statement regarding formaldehyde as a specimen preservative is

a. the nurse does not require gloves if the formaldehyde is diluted with water.
b. formaldehyde is a proven carcinogen, so the nurse always requires gloves and proper ventilation.
c. the only requirement is for the nurse to decant the formaldehyde slowly.
d. the nurse must wear goggles, gloves, and a respirator when pouring formaldehyde.

63. The preoperative RN is conducting the anesthesia consent for a patient who will be getting a peripheral nerve block. Which of the following is a potential site for a peripheral nerve block?

a. Cerebrospinal fluid (CSF).
b. Epidural space.
c. Digits.
d. Earlobe.

64. What is the color of an air hose on an anesthesia machine?

a. Green.
b. Yellow.
c. Blue.
d. White.

65. Which of the following barriers to communication almost always requires the presence of a family member or caregiver during perioperative teaching?

a. Non-English speaker.
b. Dementia.
c. Vision impairment.
d. Deafness (using sign language).

66. Which of the following is a conducting fluid distension medium that should be avoided with a monopolar active electrode?

a. Sodium chloride 0.9%
b. Mannitol 5%
c. Glycine 1.5%
d. Sorbitol 3%

67. The body part that, if incorrectly positioned, results in brachial plexus injury, is the

a. leg.
b. back.
c. arm.
d. head.

68. A perioperative nurse opened a set of special instruments onto a ring stand before surgery began, but they were untouched during this case. The appropriate action regarding these instruments following surgery is to

a. cover them for use in the next case; they were not touched and remain sterile.
b. once opened during surgery, instruments require reprocessing by CSS.
c. instruct the scrub nurse to re-wrap them and seal them with tape.
d. A and C.

69. The major concerns regarding jackknife positioning include all of the following EXCEPT

a. venous pooling in the feet and chest.
b. restricted diaphragm movement, which decreases cardiac output and ventilation.
c. increased risk of injury to the eye and ear.
d. nerve damage.

70. All of the following are risk factors for falls EXCEPT

a. a fall in previous 3 months.
b. medications.
c. impaired gait.
d. tall stature.

71. The best place to find an up-to-date protocol for sterilizing instruments that contact a CJD patient's nerve or eye tissue is the

a. Facility's Policy & Procedure Manual.
b. Centers for Disease Control and World Health Organization.
c. County Health Department.
d. State Health Department.

72. The reverse Trendelenburg position is a variation of the

a. supine position, in which the patient's head is lower than his feet.
b. prone position, in which the patient's head is higher than his feet.
c. supine position, in which the patient's head is higher than his feet.
d. lateral position, in which the patient's head rests on a pillow, level with his feet.

73. A circulating nurse on a case that requires a large amount of irrigation solution dispenses 1,000 mL of sterile NSS, and then adds 500 mL more as the case progresses. Since the circulating nurse only has 1,000 mL screw-top containers, the correct way to handle the 500 mL excess saline is to

a. replace the cap and save it for adding later.
b. leave the cap off and save it for adding later.
c. save it by handing the scrub nurse an additional bowl and pouring the remainder in it.
d. discard it; once poured, the saline is contaminated.

74. The best definition of "surgical gut" is a

a. type of nonabsorbable suture.
b. suture made from the intestines of a cat.
c. suture derived from the collagen of the submucosal layer of sheep, cattle, or hog intestine.
d. suture made from nylon.

75. The infectious bacteria usually transferred to a wound from hair is

a. *Streptococcus.*
b. *Staphylococcus.*
c. MRSA.
d. *E-coli.*

76. The person responsible for marking the surgical site is the

a. patient.
b. perioperative nurse.
c. surgeon.
d. anesthesiologist.

77. Which of the following statements are NOT true regarding silk sutures?

a. Silk sutures are thread from silkworm larvae cocoons.
b. Silk suture strands are twisted or braided.
c. Silk sutures are absorbable after a short period of time.
d. Silk sutures are commonly used for soft tissue approximation.

78. The Braden Scale for risk of developing pressure injuries assesses the following six areas: sensory perception, moisture, activity, mobility, usual nutrition pattern, and

a. friction and shear.
b. mental status.
c. pain level.
d. risk of fall.

79. The best method to prevent a patient's exhaled anesthetic gases from contaminating the OR's atmosphere is a

a. CO_2 system.
b. scavenger system connected to a suction line.
c. filtration system.
d. reservoir bag.

80. To prevent VTE during the intraoperative and immediate postoperative period, intermittent pneumatic compression devices should remain on patients daily for a minimum of:

a. 8 hours
b. 12 hours
c. 18 hours
d. 20 hours

81. The items the nurse collects to treat malignant hyperthermia include all of the following EXCEPT

a. thirty-six or more vials of Dantrolene sodium (Dantrium); enough preservative-free sterile injectable water to reconstitute the Dantrium.
b. a protocol sheet for reference; cold sterile NSS for wound irrigation; cold IV solution; ice or a cooling blanket for surface cooling; cold gastric and rectal lavage equipment; a new anesthesia circuit and carbon dioxide absorbent; and Vacutainer blood tubes for specimen testing.
c. a warming blanket; sequential stockings; warm NSS; warm IV solutions; a new anesthesia machine or circuits and carbon dioxide absorbent.
d. sodium bicarbonate; and a new anesthesia machine, if possible.

82. When educating a patient about disease management, the first step is to

a. assess the patient's knowledge level regarding the disease.
b. provide preparatory literature (e.g., pamphlets).
c. ask what the patient wants to know.
d. provide an overview.

83. The appropriate safety precaution for unscrubbed personnel working in a sterile setup is to

a. never walk between sterile fields.
b. keep a short distance from sterile fields.
c. keep their back to sterile fields.
d. wear a mask to allow proximity to sterile fields.

84. In an active shooter situation, the three actions that staff members should be taught to choose in order to survive are

a. run, hide, or fight.
b. barricade, hide, or fight.
c. confront, attack, or hide.
d. yell, run, or hide.

85. The process that kills pathogenic microorganisms through the application of liquid chemical germicides is

a. sterilization.
b. disinfection.
c. purification.
d. fumigation.

86. An example of a cost-saving technique is

a. efficient turn-over of the Operating Room between cases.
b. staff skipping breaks, except for lunch.
c. reusing laser glasses, even if they are scratched.
d. recapping sterile NSS irrigation for reuse in other cases.

87. The correct procedure for dealing with an impaired perioperative nurse is

a. advise the nurse to take sick leave and treat cause of impairment.
b. fire the nurse immediately.
c. refer the nurse to rehabilitation program and place on administrative leave.
d. follow procedures established by the state board of nursing.

88. A patient has developed a coccygeal pressure injury that is covered with a 2 × 3 cm area of black eschar with erythematous tissue around the perimeter. According to the National Pressure Injury Advisory Panel staging system, how is this pressure injury staged?

a. Stage 2.
b. Stage 3.
c. Stage 4.
d. Unstageable.

89. The circulating RN should be aware that an intravascular injection of local anesthesia from a peripheral nerve block can lead to which of the following?

a. Overdose and possible cardiac arrest.
b. Numbness.
c. Loss of the limb.
d. Paralysis of the limb.

90. When taking a telephone order, the nurse must

a. ask a second nurse to listen to the order.
b. read back the order.
c. record the order for playback.
d. ask the physician to repeat each order two times.

91. The purpose of a Veress needle insertion during a laparoscopic cholecystectomy is

a. to anesthetize the patient's skin.
b. to inject CO_2 gas into the patient's abdominal cavity.
c. to irrigate the patient's abdomen.
d. to remove excess bile from the patient.

92. All of the following are essential components of hand-off communication EXCEPT

a. effective communication techniques.
b. standardized reporting techniques.
c. use of approved abbreviations only.
d. computerized communication system.

93. The perioperative nurse should anticipate positioning equipment needed for

a. obese patients.
b. debilitated patients.
c. all patients.
d. disabled patients.

94. When opening a sterile wrapper, the flap that is opened first is the

a. distal (top) flap.
b. proximal (bottom) flap.
c. right flap.
d. left flap.

95. The food or drink that a GI patient must avoid for the first three weeks post-operatively is

a. citrus fruits.
b. green vegetables.
c. carbonated beverages.
d. dairy products.

96. A perioperative nurse drops a unique instrument needed to complete the surgery in progress. The best response by the circulating nurse is to

a. don gloves; retrieve the instrument; sanitize it; flash sterilize it; return it to the scrub nurse.
b. call area hospitals; borrow a similar instrument that is sterile; re-schedule the surgery.
c. retrieve the instrument with a sterile towel; send it to Central Sterile Supply for processing; return it to the scrub nurse.
d. don gloves; retrieve the instrument; soak it in alcohol for 5 minutes; return it to the scrub nurse.

97. A patient is being transitioned from unfractionated heparin to warfarin. Patients usually require overlapping therapy for __________ before achieving an international normalized ratio (INR, which measures how quickly blot clots) in a therapeutic range.

a. 1 day
b. 2 days
c. 2–4 days
d. 4–5 days

98. Which of the following conditions do NOT require a perioperative nurse to change the dispersive electrode (Bovie pad) site?

a. Scar tissue or excessive adipose tissue.
b. Bony prominence, pacemaker, or automatic cardiac defibrillator.
c. Abundant muscle tissue or tanned skin.
d. A metal prosthetic implant.

99. A synonym for *bariatric surgery* is

a. gall bladder surgery.
b. weight reduction surgery.
c. surgery on the elderly.
d. surgery on the pancreas.

100. The following should not be used to reduce pressure, as it may increase friction injuries

a. rolled towels.
b. convoluted foam mattress overlay.
c. foam pads.
d. viscoelastic overlay.

101. The correct safety precautions for laser use include all of the following EXCEPT

a. keeping the laser on 'ready' at all times.
b. positioning wet towels around the patient's incision site.
c. using non-reflective instruments to avoid arcing.
d. placing the laser on 'standby' when it is not in use.

102. Under the Spaulding criteria for disinfection/sterilization, semicritical items include

a. surgical instruments.
b. urinary catheters.
c. blood pressure cuffs.
d. anesthesia equipment.

103. A perioperative nurse positions her Mayo stand over the patient and prepares to pass instruments to the surgeon. The surgeon, who is very tall, instructs the anesthetist to raise the operating table. The most appropriate action is to

a. request a step stool, so she can view the surgical field clearly, and raise the stand to avoid injuring the patient.
b. move her Mayo stand to the foot of the operating table.
c. remind the surgeon that the Mayo stand should not be moved from where it is originally placed.
d. allow the anesthetist to move the Mayo stand, and adjust accordingly.

104. A patient is a surgical technologist, so as a safety precaution the perioperative nurse must ask all of the following questions EXCEPT

a. "What type of gloves do you use in the OR?"
b. "Have you ever noticed a rash after removing latex gloves?"
c. "Do you have an area of specialization in the OR?"
d. "Do you have any food allergies?"

105. The most likely nursing diagnosis for a patient who experiences slightly elevated pulse, blood pressure, and respiratory rate while in the Holding Area is

a. hypertension.
b. COPD.
c. anxiety.
d. heart disease.

106. Semi-restricted areas include

a. operating rooms.
b. procedure rooms.
c. entrance to surgical suite.
d. sterile supply storage area.

107. The appropriate action for a member of the scrub team whose glove is contaminated is to

a. step away from the sterile field, have the circulating nurse remove the contaminated glove, and don sterile gloves.
b. step away from the sterile field, have the circulating nurse remove the contaminated glove and gown, then don a sterile gown and gloves.
c. leave the sterile area, scrub, then don a sterile gown and gloves.
d. step away from sterile field, and don a sterile glove over the contaminated glove.

108. What is the most commonly used passive drain?

a. Jackson Pratt.
b. Penrose.
c. Hemovac.
d. Sump.

109. The proper use of skin staples is to

a. press the stapler firmly against the incision line.
b. "kiss" the skin gently with the stapler when applying skin staples.
c. place the staples ½ inch apart.
d. A and C.

110. The most appropriate needle for tissue that is difficult to penetrate is

a. taper-point.
b. cutting-point.
c. blunt-tip.
d. saber-tip.

111. The major reason contributing to nurses leaving their profession is

a. infectious disease exposure.
b. early work hours.
c. workplace occupational hazards.
d. difficult surgeons.

112. "The systematic, meticulous process used to identify an issue, to gather and assess the best evidence, to draft and employ a practice change, and to evaluate the process" defines

a. evidence-based practice.
b. advanced nursing practice.
c. quality-assurance practice.
d. risk-reduction practice.

113. The first step for the committee to choose new sterile drapes for the OR is to

a. compare drape costs from one manufacturer to another.
b. establish requirements for the new drapes.
c. call at least three manufacturer's sales representatives to set up demonstrations.
d. check the material for fire resistance and thickness.

114. The anesthesiologist asks the circulating nurse to perform the Sellick maneuver, which means the nurse must

a. hold the patient's hand during induction.
b. open the endotracheal tube and hand it to the anesthesiologist.
c. press on the patient's cricoid cartilage.
d. lift the patient's shoulders.

115. The psychosocial attribute important to a patient's comprehension of the procedure is

a. temperature, pulse, and respiration.
b. cultural beliefs regarding surgery.
c. skin appearance.
d. level of consciousness.

116. The nurse's first and foremost action when a fire engulfs the surgical patient's drapes is to

a. get the fire extinguisher.
b. sound the fire alarm.
c. remove the drapes from the patient.
d. announce "Code Red."

117. The most widely used method of skin surface warming to prevent hypothermia is

a. circulating water garments.
b. warming IV fluids.
c. increasing ambient temperature.
d. forced air warming.

118. The oldest, safest, least expensive, and best understood sterilization method is

a. ethylene oxide.
b. steam.
c. dry heat.
d. hydrogen peroxide gas plasma.

119. Which gloving technique poses the greatest risk of contamination to the scrub nurse?

a. Closed technique.
b. Open technique.
c. Gloved by other scrub personnel.
d. Double gloving.

120. The relevant information that the Holding Area nurse must relay to the OR nurse include all of the following EXCEPT

a. the patient has a grass allergy.
b. the patient's right leg is paralyzed.
c. the patient has a pacemaker implant.
d. the patient stated, "My brother had a really bad reaction to anesthesia in a surgery last year."

121. The competency that is NOT a minimum qualification for an OR supervisor is/are

a. managerial skills.
b. clinical expertise.
c. Central Sterilization techniques expertise.
d. interpersonal skills.

122. All of the following are good questioning techniques for interviews EXCEPT

a. information questions (who, what, when, where, how).
b. yes/no questions (Do you have headaches?).
c. clarifying questions (How long were you hospitalized?).
d. providing lists of options (throbbing, stabbing, dull).

123. Which of the following documents should be reviewed in the preprocedure assessment to verify the procedure?

a. Patient's surgical consent form
b. Patient's insurance information
c. Advance directive
d. Medication record

124. The best response to a new perioperative nurse wearing pink nail polish while scrubbing is to

a. explain to her that she must remove her nail polish prior to scrubbing.
b. do nothing; the nail polish does not pose a problem.
c. report her to the supervisor for wearing nail polish.
d. replace her with someone who has no nail polish.

125. With the traditional surgical wound classification system, a surgical wound that enters into a colonized area of the body, such as the respiratory or urinary tract, is classified as

a. Class I.
b. Class II.
c. Class III.
d. Class IV.

126. In order to prevent patient injury during surgery, when placing a patient in the lithotomy position, what should the perioperative nurse NOT do?

a. Lift the patient's legs slowly.
b. Lift only one of the patient's legs at time.
c. Lift both of the patient's legs in unison.
d. Secure the legs in leg supports.

127. The best time to schedule surgery for a patient who is infected with a known airborne-transmitted disease is

a. first case in the morning.
b. any time.
c. last case of the day.
d. do not schedule, until this patient is disease-free.

128. What is the most likely injury to result from faulty positioning that impairs blood-flow to the patient's legs?

a. Phlebothrombosis.
b. Shearing.
c. Air embolism.
d. Bronchial spasm.

129. The most appropriate responses to a patient's adverse reaction to local anesthetic is to do all of the following EXCEPT

a. inform the surgeon; establish and maintain an airway; and administer O_2.
b. ask the anesthesiologist for assistance.
c. administer Narcan.
d. administer a sedative and bring the Crash Cart

130. In the case in which a patient was not NPO prior to surgery, the perioperative nurse should have all of the following items standing by for emesis EXCEPT

a. a nasogastric tube.
b. a suction catheter with a soft tip.
c. a sterile towel.
d. an emesis basin.

131. The areas of a sterile gown that are contaminated after donning are the

a. cuffs, sleeves above the elbow, and panels below the waist.
b. panels below the waist, back, and lower arms.
c. neckline, shoulder, cuffs, and axillae (underarms).
d. cuffs to 2" above the elbow, cuffs, neckline, and axillae (underarms).

132. The team members who sign the Perioperative Report to verify that the sponge, sharps, and instrument counts were correct are

a. the surgeon and the circulating nurse.
b. the scrub nurse and the circulating nurse.
c. the anesthetist and circulating nurse.
d. the scrub technician and the scrub nurse.

133. All of the following factors increase the surgical patient's risk of infection EXCEPT

a. obesity.
b. previous joint replacement.
c. radiation therapy.
d. the administration of immunosuppressants post-operatively.

134. An older patient who has taken corticosteroids to control chronic obstructive pulmonary disease has developed a skin tear with a partial-thickness injury and an approximate 20% loss of the epidermal flap. According to the Payne–Martin Classification for Skin Tears, this is classified as

a. category I.
b. category II.
c. category III.
d. category IV.

135. A patient is eight months pregnant. Her surgery requires a supine position. How must the perioperative nurse best prevent hypotension from uterine pressure on her aorta and vena cava?

a. Raise the patient's legs onto pillows to prevent venous pooling.
b. Place a padded wedge under her right side.
c. Place a small pillow under her waist.
d. Apply sequential compression stockings to her lower legs.

136. All of the following are items that the nurse must count at the close of surgery EXCEPT

a. Kittner dissectors, lap sponges (pads), 4" x 4" RAY-TEC® (x-ray detectable) sponges.
b. gauze peanuts and tonsil sponges.
c. thrombin-soaked gelatin sponges.
d. cottonoid patties (neuro sponges).

137. The TRUE statement regarding thrombin for hemostasis is

a. thrombin is derived from porcine pancreas and controls capillary bleeding.
b. mix thrombin just prior to use because it loses potency after 20 minutes.
c. thrombin is a dry white powder, reconstituted with saline or water, and combined with oxidized cellulose.
d. bovine-derived thrombin can trigger an autoimmune response, resulting in a hemorrhage.

138. If a burn extends through the dermis and results in large watery blisters and erythema, this is classified as a

a. first-degree burn.
b. second-degree burn.
c. third-degree burn.
d. fourth-degree burn.

139. The special care requirements for ophthalmic instruments is to

a. gently hand wash them.
b. closely examine their tips after use.
c. send them to CSS for processing.
d. wash in a sterilizing machine to prevent damage from hand contact.

140. As a perioperative nurse transports his Gynecology patient out of the OR after a procedure, the drainage bag from the patient's indwelling catheter detaches from the cart and drops to the floor. The best reaction is to

a. reattach the drainage bag to a lower section of the cart.
b. place the drainage bag on the patient's abdomen temporarily, until the nurse can get to the Post Anesthesia Care Unit.
c. clamp her catheter, detach the drainage bag, and finish the transport.
d. clamp the drainage bag tubing, place the bag on top of the patient, and transport her.

141. The correct rule for performing a surgical prep is to

a. start cleaning at the dirtiest area first to allow the prep solution time to kill the bacteria.
b. start cleaning at the incision area first, then prep in circles radiating outward.
c. start cleaning at the patient's midline, then prep outward toward the extremities.
d. none of the above.

142. A perioperative nurse scrubs-in on an emergency case. In the rush to set up, the circulating nurse opens sterile 3" x 3" sponges onto the perioperative nurse's back table. The best response is to

a. count the 3" x 3" sponges and keep them as is on the back table.
b. count the 3" x 3" sponges and use them to control hemorrhaging.
c. discard the 3" x 3" sponges, so they will not be confused with radiopaque 4" x 4" sponges.
d. count the 3" x 3" sponges and use them on sponge sticks.

143. A patient undergoing emergency abdominal surgery received recent radiation of the chest. The skin in the irradiated area is dry, itchy, and scaly, and there is partial epidermal sloughing. This is categorized as a ___________ radiation burn.

a. grade I
b. grade II
c. grade III
d. grade IV

144. The surgical patients who are NOT at high-risk for developing Methicillin-Resistant Staphylococcus Aureus (MRSA) are

a. high-risk patients with underlying diseases.
b. patients with prolonged hospitalizations.
c. patients from the Intensive Care Unit.
d. patients from the Same Day Surgery unit.

145. The additional responsibility of a registered nurse while monitoring a moderately sedated patient, or one who received analgesia, is

a. the monitoring nurse should have no other responsibility that would distract from the monitors or from the patient.
b. circulating, providing the nurse can see all the monitors.
c. the monitoring nurse can scrub in, providing all the monitors are visible from the field.
d. the monitoring nurse records the surgery, to help the circulating nurse.

146. The most appropriate disinfectant to use in the OR prior to the first surgery of the day is

a. alcohol.
b. formalin.
c. hospital-grade disinfectant approved by the EPA.
d. immerse in 1N Sodium hydroxide (NaOH) in a covered pan for one hour, steam autoclave for 30 minutes at 121 °C, AND subject to routine sterilization.

147. The FALSE statement regarding an ultrasonic scalpel is

a. an ultrasonic scalpel vibrates 55,000 times per second.
b. increasing power to the ultrasonic scalpel boosts its cutting and coagulating ability.
c. an ultrasonic scalpel cuts and coagulates simultaneously.
d. an ultrasonic scalpel denatures protein to create a sticky coagulant.

148. Which of the following is an example of a neurovascular assessment that may be performed in the preoperative setting prior to the surgical procedure?

a. Nausea level.
b. Pain level.
c. Skin breakdown.
d. Peripheral pulses.

149. The decisions that are included in the nurse's Five Rights of Delegation include all of the following EXCEPT

a. right task and right circumstances.
b. right communication and right supervision.
c. right diagnosis and right status.
d. right person.

150. The most probable nursing diagnosis for a patient receiving local anesthetic, who complains of dizziness, tremors, and visual disturbances, is

a. epilepsy.
b. toxic reaction to local anesthetic.
c. hypoglycemia from NPO order.
d. excessively bright overhead lights.

151. The most common cause of delayed surgical wound healing is

a. diabetes.
b. surgical site infection (SSI).
c. malnutrition.
d. impaired circulation.

152. When using lasers during surgery, the smoke evacuation suction tube should be held

a. 1 inch from tissue interaction site.
b. 2-4 inches from tissue interaction site.
c. 4-8 inches from tissue interaction site.
d. 8-12 inches from tissue interaction site.

153. The medication identification requirement for the scrub nurse is

a. use pre-printed medication labels, or label drugs with a sterile marker when labels are unavailable.
b. store drugs in different types of containers to simplify identification.
c. when pre-printed labels are unavailable, use color-coded containers.
d. use permanent markers to label all medications.

154. The anesthesia care provider tells the circulating nurse during a cardiac surgery that she will be performing a transesophageal echocardiography (TEE). What is the primary purpose of this procedure?

a. To monitor wedge pressures.
b. To monitor myocardial ischemia.
c. To monitor myocardial infarction.
d. To evaluate esophageal tears.

155. A metal implant in a patient's right hip means the perioperative nurse must place the dispersive electrode

a. to avoid putting the metal implant in the circuit path.
b. on an extra-large dispersive electrode pad.
c. on his right thigh.
d. so that the metal implant is between the active electrode and the dispersive electrode pad.

156. The correct definition for a clean contaminated surgical wound is

a. an incision that does not pierce the GI, respiratory, or GU tracts.
b. an incision that pierces the GI, respiratory, or GU tracts by controlled means.
c. a surgical site that contains infected or dead tissue.
d. an incision that is grossly contaminated, but with no sign of infection.

157. The nurse's role in assisting the anesthesiologist during intubation is to

a. pull downwardly on the corner of the patient's mouth to enhance visualization of the vocal cords.
b. inflate the balloon on the endotracheal tube with 1 mL of air.
c. hold the endotracheal tube for easy access by the anesthesiologist.
d. apply pressure to the chin to enhance chord exposure.

158. To activate the fire extinguisher, the nurse must do all of the following EXCEPT

a. pull the pin.
b. squeeze the handle.
c. start the spray at the top of the fire, and sweep it downward.
d. focus the spray at the base of the fire.

159. The anesthesia care provider plans to perform an intercostal block during thoracic surgery. Which of the following is a potential complication of an intercostal nerve block?

a. Air embolism.
b. Numbness.
c. Headache.
d. Horner syndrome.

160. Which one of the following organizations is focused specifically on perioperative nursing?

a. AMSM.
b. IFPN.
c. AASNP.
d. AORN.

161. Which of the following is NOT true regarding shearing injuries in the OR?

a. Shearing occurs when the patient's skin remains stationary and the tissue beneath it shifts.
b. Shearing occurs when perioperative personnel pull a patient, rather than lift him.
c. Shearing occurs when the nurse inadequately pads the patient's bony prominences.
d. Shearing injuries may result in pressure injuries over time.

162. A patient with a T2 spinal cord injury develops autonomic dysreflexia, which is unrelieved by placing the patient in high Fowler's position and loosening the clothing. The next step is to

a. assess the skin for pressure areas.
b. administer antihypertensives.
c. assess bowel function.
d. assess bladder function.

163. The major advantage of laparoscopic surgery is

a. a reduced infection risk for the patient.
b. the surgeon's increased capacity to inspect the patient's abdomen.
c. the patient's reduced potential for DVT.
d. the patient's decreased venous return.

164. Which of the following is NOT a primary purpose of a "time out" immediately before beginning a surgical procedure?

a. give the staff a break before beginning the surgery.
b. verify the correct patient, procedure and site.
c. confirm the availability of surgical implants, if applicable.
d. ensure the entire surgical team is on the same page and prepared for surgery.

165. The necessary precaution the nurse must take when lowering the patient's legs from the lithotomy position is to do all of the following EXCEPT

a. extend the patient's legs completely, to prevent hip abduction.
b. lower the patient's legs quickly, to reduce back strain.
c. lower the patient's legs slowly, to prevent severe hypotension.
d. lowering the legs slowly, bending at the knees to prevent injury.

166. The best instruction to give a student nurse who placed the sterile drape on the operative area, when noticing it slid down several inches, is

a. "Reposition the drape over the incision site and continue draping."
b. "Discard that drape and ask the circulating nurse for a new one."
c. "Remove the contaminated drape and place it on the back table."
d. "Tell the circulating nurse to re-prep the surgical area, and then drape it again with sterile material."

167. Which of the following complications are specific to arteriovenous (AV) fistula patients postoperatively?

a. Paralysis.
b. Renal failure.
c. Stroke.
d. Hemorrhage at the surgical site.

168. A patient's medical record indicates that a patient is a male named Robert; however, the patient wears makeup and typically feminine clothing. How should the nurse address this patient?

a. Ask the patient if he is transgender.
b. Ask the patient what pronouns are preferred.
c. Address the patient as any other male.
d. Address the patient as any other female.

169. Before applying alcohol in an alcohol-based surgical hand scrub, the person should

a. rinse hands and forearms with water and dry.
b. wash hands and forearms with antimicrobial soap and dry thoroughly.
c. wash hands and forearms with non-antimicrobial soap and dry thoroughly.
d. complete a 2-minute scrub with antimicrobial soap and hand brush.

170. The TRUE statement regarding lasers is

a. carbon dioxide (CO_2) lasers cannot damage the cornea.
b. argon lasers can damage the cornea.
c. Neodymium-Yttrium-Aluminum-Garnet (Nd:YAG) lasers can damage the retina.
d. optical damage occurs with carbon dioxide (CO_2) lasers only.

171. Which of the following are types of retractors?

a. Richardson, Army-Navy, and Deaver.
b. Allis, Babcock, and Kocher.
c. Towel clip and sponge forceps.
d. Castroviejo, Metzenbaum, and Mayo.

172. A perioperative nurse is interviewing a patient preoperatively who is having an exploratory laparotomy for abdominal pain. In her surgical history, the nurse notes that she had an adjustable gastric band placed three years ago. Which of the following is a complication specific to these procedures that might be contributing to her condition?

a. Incisional hernia formation.
b. Anastomosis leakage.
c. Tissue erosion.
d. Anastomotic stricture.

173. Which of the following is a triggering agent for malignant hyperthermia?

a. Halothane.
b. Nitrous oxide.
c. Ketamine.
d. Propofol.

174. Which is the weak anesthesia gas that supplements other inhalation agents and narcotics?

a. Isoflurane.
b. Desflurane.
c. Nitrous oxide.
d. Sevoflurane.

175. The proper procedure for attaching a blade to a scalpel handle is to

a. grasp the blade firmly between the index finger and thumb, then attach the blade to the handle.
b. use a needle holder to attach the blade to the handle.
c. open the blade package, but leave its sharp end covered while attaching its blunt end to the handle, then remove the package completely.
d. grasp the blade with toothed forceps and attach it to the handle.

176. Which one of the following is an example of a mass casualty event as opposed to a mass effect event?

a. Hurricane.
b. Pandemic.
c. Flood.
d. Earthquake.

177. The maximum insufflation pressure during a laparoscopic cholecystectomy is

a. 10 mmHg.
b. 21 mmHg.
c. 15 mmHg.
d. 12 mmHg.

178. A perioperative nurse scrubs according to hospital protocol, then accidentally touches the faucet with her hand while rinsing. Her most appropriate next step is to

a. proceed into the OR.
b. rinse for an extra minute, and then proceed to the OR.
c. start her scrub over from the beginning, using a new scrub sponge/brush.
d. wear double gloves on her contaminated hand, and proceed to the OR.

179. The appropriate method for transferring a patient from a stretcher onto an operating table is to

a. lock the stretcher's wheels prior to moving the patient; the OR table is always locked, so do not check it.
b. enlist at least two people for transfer: one to stabilize the stretcher, and one on the opposite side of the operating table to receive the patient.
c. if the patient is awake, there is no need for a second person to receive him or her.
d. raise the stretcher higher than the operating table, so the patient can move down onto the operating table independently.

180. The appropriate safety precautions when working with methyl methacrylate include all of the following EXCEPT

a. do not wear contact lenses.
b. do not use electronic equipment while mixing.
c. pour the powder into the liquid.
d. wear a face shield and double gloves.

181. Which of the following traits is NOT an advantage of steam sterilization?

a. Readily available.
b. Leaves no toxic residue.
c. Compatible with all materials.
d. Fast.

182. Performance improvement efforts attempt to do all of the following EXCEPT

a. improve quality.
b. improve effectiveness.
c. increase the number of positive surgical outcomes.
d. manage costs.

183. Indications of transurethral resection syndrome associated with intra- or extravasation of irrigation fluids include:

a. hypertension
b. hypernatremia
c. abdominal pain
d. bradycardia

184. Which of the following statements is NOT true regarding blunt-tip surgical needles?

a. The surgeon's assistant uses a blunt-tip needle for skin closure.
b. Blunt-tip needles are available in several gauges.
c. Blunt-tip needles are for internal suturing.
d. Blunt-tip needles prevent percutaneous injuries in the OR.

185. If heat is lost when air currents move across the skin, such as from an air conditioning vent, this type of heat loss is categorized as:

a. evaporative
b. convective
c. radiant
d. conductive

186. The preferred method for shaving a male patient's abdomen prior to his surgical procedure is to

a. shave him with a razor, warm water, and antiseptic soap.
b. shave him with a razor on dry skin.
c. use electric clippers to shave his abdomen.
d. use hot wax to remove his hair.

187. The three steps of the Universal Protocol for preventing wrong site, wrong procedure, and wrong person surgery are

a. preoperative verification; mark the operative site; and take a "time out" before starting surgery.
b. assess allergies and implants; read the History for the patient's hospitalizations; and take a "time out" before taking the patient to the OR
c. mark the operative site; confirm the consent form was signed; and identify the patient.
d. check the medication history; verify the patient's identity; confirm the operative site with the surgeon.

188. The nurse should avoid wearing all of the following EXCEPT

a. artificial fingernails.
b. fingernail polish (freshly applied).
c. rings.
d. necklaces.

189. The information that the circulating nurse is NOT responsible for recording is

a. temperature of the operating room.
b. incision time.
c. end of surgery time.
d. anesthesia induction time.

190. During a transurethral prostatectomy performed with regional anesthesia, the patient's abdomen becomes rigid and swollen, the patient complains of nausea and abdominal pain and becomes hypotensive, and the nurse notes a decrease in bladder irrigating solution. The most likely cause is

a. transurethral prostatectomy syndrome.
b. bladder perforation.
c. bowel perforation.
d. internal hemorrhage.

191. Following a right total knee arthroplasty, the patient complains of throbbing pain in the right calf, and an examination shows slight edema of the calf and slight erythema of the mid-calf. These signs and symptoms are consistent with

a. infection.
b. lymphedema.
c. cellulitis.
d. deep vein thrombosis.

192. A circulating RN is caring for a patient having a ventral hernia repair. During her preoperative assessment, the nurse notices this patient is morbidly obese. Which one of the following is an associated disease with this condition?

a. Type 1 diabetes.
b. Osteoporosis.
c. GERD.
d. Hypotension.

193. Which of the following is a contraindication to intermittent pneumatic compression therapy?

a. Age >60
b. Smoking
c. Stroke
d. Pulmonary edema

194. The nurse's safety precaution steps before the surgeon uses a laser include all of the following EXCEPT

a. ensure everyone in the room wears appropriate eye protection, even for endoscopic laser procedures.
b. place a "DANGER, Laser Radiation" sign at every Procedure Room entrance or exit.
c. do not cover the window in the OR door or any other windows, since laser beams do not penetrate glass.
d. place wet gauze pads on the anesthetized patient's eyes.

195. Most OR fires that injure the patient occur in the

a. abdominal area, from electrosurgery sparks.
b. facial area, due to its high oxygen concentration.
c. intra-abdominal area during laparoscopic laser usage.
d. perineal area, from electrosurgery or laser usage.

196. An 82-year-old patient suffered a fractured hip during a fall. The patient, who had seemed alert, exhibits sudden fluctuating changes in consciousness with language disturbance, disorientation, confusion, and audiovisual hallucinations. The patient should be assessed for

a. traumatic brain injury.
b. delirium.
c. stroke.
d. dementia.

197. The best location to shave a patient so that his hair removal occurs as close to the time of surgery as possible is

a. in the OR, as part of the prep.
b. in the Holding Area.
c. in the patient's hospital room.
d. in the hallway outside the OR.

198. Symptoms of bone cement implantation syndrome (BCIS) include

a. vasoconstriction and hypertension.
b. unstable prosthesis.
c. erythema and swelling around prosthesis site.
d. pulmonary hypertension.

199. The best method for transferring contaminated instruments to Central Sterile Supply (CSS) is to

a. transport contaminated instruments sealed in a closed container, cart, or plastic bag.
b. transport contaminated instruments on an open cart.
c. transport contaminated instruments in a large basin, submerged in water.
d. transport contaminated instruments covered in a used drape.

200. The scrub nurse's duty when receiving sponges, sharps or sutures with needles is to

a. tell the surgeon to wait for his next instrument and immediately count these items with the circulating nurse.
b. count these items as soon as possible after receiving them, then notify the circulating nurse.
c. keep these items unopened on the back table, until there is time to open and count them with the circulating nurse.
d. put the items aside for the circulating nurse to count, and hand the surgeon his next instrument.

Answer Key and Explanations for Test #1

1. A: Sometimes an anxious, premedicated patient answers to a wrong name, or two patients have the same or similar names. The *best* method to confirm a patient's identity is to check the wristband, confirm that it matches the name and unique number on the chart, and ask the patient (or parent/guardian) to spell the name. The Holding Area nurse may assist with patient identification, but the perioperative nurse must still check the chart, the wristband, and ask the patient to say his name.

2. B: Position the table strap 2 inches *above* the knees as soon as the patient moves onto the operating table. Remove the strap when the patient is ready for transport to the Recovery Room, and perioperative personnel are standing beside the patient for transfer assistance.

3. B: Dust and lint that carry microorganisms settle on horizontal surfaces, therefore these surfaces require the most attention from cleaners. Nonetheless, all surfaces require attention and care to maintain a clean and sterile environment.

4. B: The perioperative nurse should *never* attempt to sterilize a single-use item. The manufacturer must meet extremely stringent requirements for preparing a single-use item. If the nurse attempts to sterilize it, then the hospital assumes all liability. The nurse should phone Central Sterile Supply and send the item to them by porter. The CSS supervisor will decide if reprocessing complies with hospital policy. 2% alkaline glutaraldehyde can sterilize some items, but the immersion period is a minimum of 10 hours. The manufacturer would have to approve glutaraldehyde sterilization for this particular instrument. Inform the surgeon and anesthesiologist of the situation.

5. C: In addition to assisting the anesthetist, standing next to the patient during induction provides emotional support and prevents patient falls. The scrub nurse is responsible for observing the sterile set-up.

6. A: Head injuries may occur when the overhead lights are positioned for surgery, prior to bringing the patient to the OR, therefore staff in the OR must take care to attend to their surroundings. Fires are not a risk from overhead lights, nor is contamination. Enhanced anxiety may be caused by the overhead lights in the OR but this would not be posed until after the patient has been brought to the OR and can be managed with medication and communication.

7. A: A Bier Block involves the intravenous injection of an anesthetic agent (usually Lidocaine) into the vein of an extremity bound by two tourniquets, or a double cuffed tourniquet. Prior to inflating the tourniquets, the nurse wraps the elevated extremity with the Esmarch bandage to enhance the blood drainage. The surgeon or anesthetist injects the anesthetic agent.

8. B: Once the pointed towel clip penetrates the drape, it becomes contaminated; removing it would involve pulling it back through the drape and contaminating the sterile field. The *best* option is to re-clasp it. Ignoring the towel clip is inappropriate because it could fall and harm the patient with its sharp points. Removal of the towel clip by anyone would contaminate the sterile field.

9. C: The circulating nurse should move any foot pedal that is not in use, so the surgeon does not inadvertently step on it. 100% oxygen is not a good choice for facial surgery because it is a fire hazard. A lower percentage of oxygen or air is appropriate for most patients. Air is in the yellow tank on an anesthesia machine. Shaving a man's beard or mustache is usually unnecessary; coating the hair with a water-based lubricant prevents fire. The electrosurgery pencil belongs in a holster when it is not in use; never rest it on the drape.

10. B: Once a sterile field is set up, the perioperative staff must *continually* monitor it. A two-hour window between the opening of the sterile items and the start of surgery is acceptable. It would not be cost-effective to discard the sterile items and order new ones. The staff may leave the room *only* if someone who relieves them can continually monitor the sterile fields.

11. A: Epinephrine should be given immediately if indications of anaphylaxis are evident, followed by increased IV fluids (crystalloid) to treat hypotension. Delay in administering epinephrine correlates with increased rate of death. Albuterol per nebulizer may be administered to relieve bronchospasm. Corticosteroids do not treat the immediate reaction but may prevent the biphasic recurrence of symptoms. Antihistamines (combination H_1 and H_2 blockers) are usually given, but the onset of action is slower than epinephrine, so they do not provide immediate relief of symptoms.

12. A: If the sponge count is incorrect, inform the surgeon and anesthesiologist immediately. The patient may need to remain under anesthesia until an abdominal x-ray determines if the sponge is still inside the wound.

13. C: The AORN recommends the use of chlorhexidine gluconate (CHG) as a cleansing agent during the patient's preoperative shower. CHG significantly inhibits the growth of *Staphylococcus epidermis,* and Gram-positive and Gram-negative bacteria, and viruses. By reducing surface skin colonization, CHG subsequently decreases the postoperative incidence of infection. Dove soap has no antibacterial properties. Povidone iodine and alcohol are often used in the OR as skin preps, but are inappropriate for showering.

14. B: During x-ray studies of the hips and femur, lead shielding should be applied to protect the ovaries or testes if possible. Lead shielding is indicated to protect the thyroid during x-ray studies above the waist, including the trunk, arms, and head. Women of childbearing age should be questioned about the possibility of pregnancy and the physician notified because x-rays pose a risk to the developing fetus. Patients should be carefully positioned so that only the necessary body part is within the radiation field.

15. A: An increase in the number of people in the OR increases the quantity of microorganisms, changes the traffic patterns of the OR due to increased number of individuals present, and increases the possibility of a surgical site infection (SSI). While this experience may improve public relations and increased interest in surgical careers, this is the least likely effect.

16. B: The most common cause of toxic anterior segment syndrome (TASS) is improper cleaning and sterilization of instruments contacting the eye, including germicide or detergent residue. Other less common causes include contaminated solutions, powder from surgical gloves, ointments, and medications. TASS can result in loss of vision because of damage of intraocular tissue. Instruments should be wiped with sterile water after use and immersed in sterile water at the end of the procedure to prevent formation of biofilms.

17. B: The perioperative nurse should immediately inform the anesthesiologist and surgeon about the possibility of malignant hyperthermia. Muscle biopsy is a diagnostic test to rule out this life-threatening, inherited condition. Telling the patient that the fever was probably due to an infection is an assumption with no supporting evidence. Informing the patient that the anesthetist will monitor his body temperature is accurate, but if the patient has a history of malignant hyperthermia, it is imperative to get a proper diagnosis prior to administering anesthesia. His body temperature is more likely to drop as a response to the cool OR, so the warm blanket may help prevent hypothermia.

18. C: Numerous factors influence surgical scheduling. Schedule infectious patients late in the day. The availability of specialty rooms, teams, and equipment are important. Surgeons usually have certain hours set aside for surgical cases. Coordinating with the surgeon's office is an important aspect of creating a schedule. The lunch schedule varies with the float nurses' availability changes, and as cases finish. Lunch breaks are an ongoing concern for the nurse who is coordinating the day's cases as they unfold.

19. A: The circulating nurse should wear gloves or use a sponge stick to handle any sponge that comes from the surgical field. Microscopic contaminants are invisible, so even if the sponge appears clean, treat it as soiled. The AORN recommends the use of clear pocketed count bags that allow for the visualization and separation of sponges. This bag should be maintained in a location that can be visualized by the surgeon. Per AORN recommendations, sponge counts should occur throughout the procedure (when new items are added to the surgical field, prior to wound closure and the closure of a cavity, any time a discrepancy occurs, and prior to any nurse/scrub technician turnover), and again during the final count with the scrub nurse/technician and the circulator.

20. B: Halon is the best fire extinguisher for the OR. The halon extinguisher is lightweight, easy to use, and versatile. Although the label of a halon extinguisher states it is effective on Class B (flammable liquids and grease) and Class C (electrical) fires, it also works on Class A (wood, cloth, paper, and most plastics).

21. C: Never use 100% oxygen (O_2) when assisting a facial surgeon because it increases the chances of a fire. Use a draping technique that does not allow pockets of O_2 to form. Oxygen that is trapped under the drape concentrates and becomes a fire hazard. Coat the patient's facial hair with a water-soluble lubricant during facial surgery, if the surgeon will employ any type of cautery, rather than trimming it which still leaves risk for facial hair to catch on fire.

22. B: Atelectasis is common following major surgical procedures because taking a deep breath and coughing can be painful. Atelectasis typically occurs on one side, although bilateral atelectasis can also occur. Patients are often asymptomatic or have mild symptoms unless the atelectasis progresses to pneumonia. Signs and symptoms may include diminished cough, reduced breath sounds, and pain in the area involved. Low-grade fever and dyspnea are common as well. Treatment may include continuous positive airway pressure, bronchodilators, chest physiotherapy, and flexible fiber-optic bronchoscopy (if obstructive).

23. C: The Army-Navy retractor is double-ended. A Weitlaner is a Balfour (self-retaining retractor) with a blade. The Army-Navy retractor does not contain a suction port.

24. B: When placing the patient into the prone position, all movements should be slow and gentle. A minimum of four people should work as a team to ensure the patient's safety. The anesthesiologist supports the head and neck and maintains the position of the endotracheal tube. The second member of the perioperative team turns the patient onto his/her side on the stretcher. The third member, positioned on the opposite side of the operating table, 'catches' the patient while supporting the chest and abdomen. A fourth person turns the patient's legs in unison. Rolling the patient independently is dangerous not only to the patient but to the nurse, and can threaten back injuries.

25. B: The appropriate technique for the circulating nurse to remove a contaminated glove from a member of the surgical team is to grasp the glove approximately 2" below the co-worker's wrist.

Carefully remove it, taking care *not* to pull down the cuff. Once the coworker's hand went through the cuff, the cuff was contaminated. The glove should not be gasped close to the co-worker's wrist.

26. C: Overhead pages can be intrusive and distracting and should be replaced by text messaging if possible, with pagers and cell phones on the silent/vibration mode or lowered ring tones for standard phones. Staff should lower voices and keep conversation to a minimum, using structured communication methods for essential information. The persons present during procedures should be limited to those who are essential. Staff members should receive education on the importance of noise reduction and posters and reminders should be displayed prominently.

27. C: A suprapubic incision is also called a Pfannenstiel. It is a gently curved, transverse incision, extending across the patient's lower abdomen, approximately 1cm above the *symphysis pubis*. Suprapubic incisions are commonly used for obstetric and gynecological procedures, such as elective Cesarean sections. The midabdominal transverse incision runs from slightly above the patient's umbilicus and extends laterally to the lumbar region. The subcostal is an oblique incision that begins in the epigastrium and extends laterally at an oblique angle, ending slightly below the patient's costal margin.

28. B: The best precaution before wrapping an Esmarch bandage around a patient's arm is to raise the patient's arm to allow for venous drainage, thereby preventing edema and necrosis later.

29. C: Fear of pain can be a strong deterrent to mobilization, so the patient's activity intolerance is likely caused by psychological factors associated with fear that she might experience a fall, like her friend did. The patient needs reassurance that efforts are made to protect against falls, such as by the use of a gait belt and walker to provide stability and support while ambulating. The patient should also collaborate in setting realistic goals for increasing her mobility.

30. A: Over pressurization during abdominal insufflation with CO_2 for a laparoscopic procedure may result in hypercarbia (not hypocarbia) as excess CO_2 diffuses into the blood. Pressure on the phrenic nerve may cause postoperative neck and shoulder pain, and pressure against the diaphragm may cause gastric regurgitation and aspiration. The reduction in intrathoracic space may cause decreased respiratory effort and cardiac output. Pressure should be constantly monitored and maintained at 14-16 mmHg.

31. B: Before anesthesia induction, the minimum prewarming time to reduce the risk of hypothermia is 10 minutes. If a patient has a low core body temperature before surgery, it is important to normalize the temperature before the patient is transferred to the operating room if possible. Prewarming patients results in higher core body temperatures during the operative procedure and higher postoperative temperatures.

32. D: Essential perioperative patient assessment includes: Allergies, especially to medications or latex; implants or pacemakers, which affect coagulation during electrocautery; and confirmation of the type and location of the proposed surgery. Age and weight are important for anesthesia, but an approximation is sufficient. *Exact* age and weight are unnecessary.

33. A: The perioperative nurse exercises active listening, and offers the patient reassurance to alleviate anxiety. All surgery carries some risk. Telling the patient that there is nothing to fear is inappropriate, as is promising the patient that everything will be ok, which can never be guaranteed. The perioperative nurse should not speak to the patient for the sake of distraction, because some patients may have questions or prefer silence as a mode to alleviate anxiety. The perioperative nurse should let the patient guide the methods utilized to communicate effectively and therapeutically.

34. C: Drapes should not be adjusted once they are placed. Drapes should be unfolded carefully rather than shaken and should not be fanned but allowed to fall in place by gravity. Any unnecessary movement should be avoided, as it may cause air migration of particles, such as lint or dust. The person draping should avoid reaching across an unsterile area while draping and should hold sterile drapes above the level of the waist. Any contaminated drape must be immediately discarded.

35. A: The *Perioperative Patient-Focused Model* emphasizes the *outcome-driven* nature of perioperative patient care. The prevention of injury, reduction of risk, and implementation of a nursing care plan are parts of this overall plan.

36. A: Making eye contact provides a connection and shows caring and involvement in the communication. Avoiding contact may indicate someone is not telling the truth or is uncomfortable, fearful, ashamed, or hiding something. People may touch themselves (lick lips, pick at skin, scratch) if they are anxious. Tapping of the foot, moving the legs, or fidgeting may indicate nervousness. Rubbing the hands together is sometimes a self-comforting measure. Mixed messages, such as fidgeting but speaking with a calm voice, may indicate uncertainty or anxiety. A high-pitched tone of voice may indicate nervousness or stress.

37. A: "Memory" refers to any material, including sutures that tends to return to its original positioning or folding position. Gently stretch the memory suture, taking care not to create tension on its swaged needle.

38. D: All staff members are responsible for identifying performance improvement projects. Performance improvement should be an ongoing process at all levels of the institution. Continuous quality process improvement begins by identifying one process that needs improvement. It might be something as small as improving paging or as large as reducing infection rates, but once a problem is identified, first steps to solve the problem are initiated. When the steps to improve one process are completed, another project is picked for improvement. In many cases, multiple continuous improvement projects may be in process at the same time.

39. D: Calcium channel blockers are contraindicated as treatment for malignant hyperthermia as they may result in severe hyperkalemia and myocardial depression. The primary treatment is 8-10 mg/kg of dantrolene sodium with repeat doses of 2.5 mg/kg up to 4 times. Other treatments include insulin in 50% glucose solution (0.15 units/kg of regular insulin in 1 mL/kg of glucose or 10 mg of regular insulin in 50 mL of glucose) and/or calcium chloride for treatment of hyperkalemia. Lidocaine or amiodarone may be indicated for cardiac arrhythmias.

40. C: The soiled gown worn during surgery is removed, after it is untied by the perioperative nurse, by grasping the gown at one shoulder seam and pulling the gown forward and inside out over the gloved hand. Then, the same procedure is followed for the other side. The gown should be held out away from the body during removal and placed in the proper container, avoiding contact with the body. The gloves are then removed, followed by the mask.

41. A: A biological indicator (BI) is a strip, ampoule, or capsule that contains live, highly resistant spores of a known type, to test the efficacy of a sterilizer. Chemical indicators contain a dye that changes color under certain conditions. Chemical indicators do not guarantee sterility, but determine that the parameters for sterilization have been met.

42. A: AORN recommends the double-glove technique for invasive surgeries. Double-gloving decreases the number of perforations of the inner glove. Not all invasive surgeries require an x-ray apron, high booties, or a laser high-filtration mask.

43. A: If a fiber-optic cord or connector detaches during use, the heat may result in a drape fire. Never place *uncoupled* cords on the patient's drapes. Remove fiber-optic headlights when the physician finishes with them, to eliminate the possibility of igniting surgical gowns or clothing.

44. B: Anesthetic agents, such as halothane and isoflurane, rarely cause anaphylactic reactions. Most anaphylaxis relates to antibiotics (penicillin, cephalosporins, sulfonamides) or latex. Isosulfan blue 1% (a blue dye) results in severe allergic reactions or anaphylaxis in up to 3% of those receiving the dye, commonly used for sentinel node biopsies. Typically, with IgE-mediated response (anaphylactic shock), an antigen triggers release of substances, such as histamine and prostaglandins, which affect the skin, cardiopulmonary, and GI systems. Each time the person has contact with the antigen, more antibodies form in response, so allergic reactions worsen with each contact.

45. A: The SBAR communication process includes:

- (S) Situation: Description of the situation, including a brief statement of the problem, as well as identifying ward/unit, patient's name and room number, and self.
- (B) Background: All pertinent information regarding the problem, including diagnosis, admission date, current medications, treatments (including IV fluids), vital signs, laboratory findings, and code status (DNR).
- (A) Assessment: Opinion of the situation from nurse's perspective.
- (R) Recommendation: Patient needs (physician orders, physician visit, and laboratory tests).

46. A: Clinically significant hyponatremia may occur during some surgeries and procedures (transurethral prostatic resection, cystoscopy) because of intravasation of fluids. Normal value is 135-145 mEq/L with hyponatremia less than 135 and hypernatremia greater than 145. Sodium (Na) regulates fluid volume, osmolality, acid-base balance, and activity in the muscles, nerves, and myocardium. It is the primary cation (positive ion) in extracellular fluid (ECF), necessary to maintain ECF levels that are needed for tissue perfusion. Indications of hyponatremia include:

- Hypertension initially followed by hypotension
- Nausea and vomiting
- Bradycardia
- Irritability, lethargy, and alterations in consciousness
- Cerebral edema with seizures and coma
- Dyspnea to respiratory failure

47. D: During the turnover between patients, floor cleaning should include 3- to 4-foot perimeter around operating table and visibly soiled areas. Protocol in dealing with hazardous wastes, such as blood and body fluids, must be followed. Cleaning the entire floor is not necessary and adds to turn over time, decreasing OR utilization, although it should be cleaned at the end of the day or according to scheduled protocol (usually 1 or more times daily) for operating rooms with extended hours.

48. C: The anesthetized patient may experience vomiting, laryngospasms, or bronchospasms during extubation. Hyperventilation is not a common complication during this process.

49. A: Exposure to anesthetic agents may cause miscarriages, reduced fertility, and liver, renal, and neurological diseases. Leukemia and heart disease are generally not the results of exposure to anesthetic agents.

50. D: A JP drains a surgical site of small amounts of fluid and blood, whereas the larger Hemovac is both a drain and a device for autologous retransfusion. There are other closed drains that prevent wound contamination, such as the Stryker Constavac. Neither JP nor Hemovac attach to external suction, lie flat, nor contain double-lumens. JP drains are used to remove small amounts of pus, infectious fluid, and blood. The larger reservoir attached to Hemovac drain allows for accurate measurement of drainage, so it can be retained and reinfused to minimize the patient's blood loss.

51. A: The nurse should call for an adult medical translator. Patients may bring family members, often children, to translate, but this is not a good solution as children often lack the maturity to assume this responsibility and may also lack the vocabulary or understanding to translate effectively, leading to serious misunderstandings. Interpreters should have training in medical vocabulary, so simply choosing any speaker of the target language, such as a housekeeper, is not good practice.

52. C: Malignant hyperthermia (MH) is not associated with a thin physique and underdeveloped muscles. Those who are susceptible to malignant hyperthermia often exhibit large, strong muscles and/or obesity, and may have a history of unexplained fevers, heat stroke, or family history of death after surgery. MH is more common in males, especially those younger than 18 years, and is also associated with central core diseases, such as neuromuscular disorders, including Duchenne muscular dystrophy. All patients should be screened for risk factors for MH prior to surgery so triggering agents can be avoided.

53. B: When electrosurgery or laser use results in surgical smoke, evacuate the smoke (plume) with suction that has an in-line filter. If a large amount of smoke is present, a free-standing smoke evacuator is required. Use a laser mask (with high particle filtration) to prevent air-borne contaminants from entering the respiratory systems of the perioperative staff. Never leave the OR doors open during any surgical procedure.

54. B: Begin counting with the sponges that are on the surgical field, sponge sticks, Mayo stand, and then the back table. The circulating nurse watches and confirms the count with the scrub nurse, completing the count with the soiled sponges. The final number must be the same as the number of sponges opened for the case.

55. C: Standard 12: Ethics from the Standards of Perioperative Nursing requires that the nurse maintain professional and therapeutic boundaries. The nurse should make arrangements for a different nurse to complete the assessment because the nurse may have biases or preconceived ideas about the patient that may interfere with an accurate assessment and evaluation. The patient may not have shared personal information with the nurse and may feel uncomfortable answering personal questions; however, the patient may not want to offend the nurse by objecting.

56. C: When encountering another person who is "scrubbed in," pass back-to-back. The back is not considered sterile, so do not turn the back to the OR table. Back-to-back is the best technique for passing.

57. B: Both the circulating nurse and the scrub nurse *must* witness the sponge count. The circulating nurse should quickly count with the scrub nurse, and then relay the message.

58. C: Frequent, prolonged exposure to anesthetic gases in the OR presents a serious health threat to perioperative staff. Beware of dizziness, nausea, headaches, fatigue, drowsiness, and decreased mental acuity in oneself or one's teammates. Hyperactivity, diaphoresis, and decreased body temperature are not characteristic signs or symptoms of exhaled anesthetic gas in the OR.

59. A: Dispersive electrode pads are *not* interchangeable. Call for one that matches the machine, and if unavailable, exchange the machine for one that matches the pad. A hand-held cauterizer is suitable for minor cases, but is inappropriate for major surgeries. The dispersive electrode is useless if not attached to the correct generator.

60. A: Prophylactic medications, such as antibiotics, are usually administered within 30 minutes to 1 hour of surgery, according to specific guidelines for the type of procedure. Antibiotic prophylaxis is routinely given for high-risk procedures (e.g., cardiac surgery) or high-risk individuals (e.g., immunocompromised, elderly, obese, diabetic). In some cases, prophylaxis is given prior to the procedure and immediately after. Guidelines should specify the type of procedure requiring prophylaxis, the time and route of administration, and the person responsible for administration.

61. B: Cardiac output (CO) is determined by the heart rate (HR) times the stroke volume (SV). Stroke volume is the amount of blood returned from the heart after each contraction. The equation commonly used to represent this is $CO = HR \times SV$.

62. B: Formaldehyde is a proven carcinogen and a respiratory irritant that also causes watering of the eyes. Formaldehyde can fix contact lenses to the wearer's eyes. Perioperative nurses should wear gloves and use formaldehyde only under a fume hood, or at least in a well-ventilated area.

63. C: Cerebrospinal fluid and epidural space refer to spinal and epidural anesthesia. Digits are one of the many possible injection sites for nerve blocks. The earlobe would be an ineffective location for a peripheral nerve block.

64. B: The color code on an anesthesia machine is yellow for air, green for oxygen, and blue for nitrous oxide. Gas fittings are not interchangeable, to prevent injuries.

65. B: Dementia requires the presence of a family member or caregiver during perioperative teaching because the patient may not comprehend instructions or may not remember them. Non-English speakers and the deaf who use sign language should be provided translators. Vision impairment is not necessarily an impediment to teaching; the patient should be able to hear and respond appropriately, although the nurse may need to use more descriptions and to allow the patient to explore objects manually. In some cases, such as with procedures that require vision, family or caregivers may need to assist.

66. A: A conducting fluid distension medium that should be avoided with a monopolar active electrode is sodium chloride 0.9% because of the risk of heat transfer and injury to tissues, although it can be used with a bipolar active electrode. With monopolar electrosurgery, nonconductive media, such as mannitol 5%, glycine 1.5%, and sorbitol 3%, are used.

67. C: Improper positioning of the patient's arm (or arm board) may result in injury to the brachial plexus.

68. B: Once opened during surgery, special surgical instruments require reprocessing. These instruments should not be covered for use in the next case. Nor should the scrub nurse re-wrap them and seal them with tape.

69. C: Jackknife position is used for many proctological procedures. Jackknife is one of the most precarious positions. The patient's mean arterial blood pressure may drop, due to venous pooling in the lower extremities and chest. A decrease in cardiac output and respirations may result from the restricted diaphragm movement. Nerve damage has been a suspected risk from this position also, due to the pressure points in this position. Injury to the ear and eye are more common in the prone position.

70. D: Stature (tall or short) is not a risk factor for falls. The 3 primary factors are:

- History of fall within the previous 3 months.
- Medications: A wide range, including antihypertensives, antidepressants, diuretics, and antihistamines.
- Impaired gait: Arthritis, peripheral neuropathy, Parkinson disease, deformities, stroke, and orthopedic problems/surgery. Weakness, loss of muscle mass, and confusion may contribute to gait disorders.

Other risk factors may include older age (although some younger people may also be at risk for falls), depression, hypothyroidism, orthostatic hypotension, heart attack, and dizziness.

71. B: Prions are responsible for the transfer of CJD, an always fatal neurological disease. Prions resist routine sterilization and disinfection techniques. Protocols for sterilization of instruments following exposure to eye or neurological tissue of a CJD patient are evolving. The Center for Disease Control (CDC) and the World Health Organization (WHO) have the latest information on removing infectious prions.

72. C: The reverse Trendelenburg position is a version of the supine position, in which the patient's head rests higher than the feet.

73. D: After removing the cap of NSS irrigation fluid and dispense it onto the sterile field, discard the remainder in the bottle. Recapping is inappropriate. The top of the bottle is considered contaminated, since drops may have encountered the outside of the bottle during the primary pouring.

74. C: Surgical gut refers to suture that is derived from collagen found in the submucosal layer of the intestines of sheep, cattle, or hogs. "Catgut" is a misnomer and may come from the Arabic word *kit*, which means "dancing master's fiddle." Nylon suture is nonabsorbable.

75. B: Hair is a major source of *Staphylococcus.* The number of microorganisms found on hair correlates with the length and cleanliness of the hair.

76. C: Only the surgeon who performs the procedure marks the surgical site. This designation and responsibility is meant to minimize errors in surgical location that may arise from erroneous designation, miscommunication or lack of surgical site clarification.

77. C: Silk is prepared from thread spun by silkworm larvae. It is twisted or braided to increase its strength. Silk sutures are commonly used for soft tissue approximation. They may be absorbed after several years.

78. A: Friction and shear. Braden Scale scores are detailed as follows:

Sensory perception	(1) Completely limited, (2) very limited, (3) slightly limited, (4) no impairment
Moisture	(1) Constantly moist, (2) very moist, (3) occasionally moist, (4) rarely moist
Activity	(1) Bed, (2) chair, (3) occasional walk, (4) frequent walks
Mobility	(1) Immobile, (2) limited, (3) slightly limited, (4) no limitations

Usual nutrition pattern	(1) Very poor, (2) inadequate, (3) adequate, (4) excellent
Friction and shear	(1) Problem (skin frequently slides down the sheets and needs help to move), (2) potential problem (skin slides somewhat during moves, needs assistance), (3) no apparent problem

79. B: The anesthesia machine has a scavenger system, which connects to a suction line. This helps prevent a patient's exhaled anesthetic gases from contaminating the OR's atmosphere.

80. C: To prevent VTE during the intraoperative and immediate postoperative period, intermittent pneumatic compression devices should remain on patients for a daily minimum of 18 hours, and the wear time should be automatically recorded by the device. The sleeves must be applied correctly, and any protective stockinette or compression stockings worn under the sleeves must be free of wrinkles. Tubing attached to the device should be placed away from the patient's skin or any area in which it may result in a pressure injury.

81. C: At least 36 vials of Dantrolene sodium (Dantrium) are necessary for a 175-pound patient. Reconstitute each vial with preservative-free sterile injectable water, and shake vigorously to achieve adequate mixing. Treat acidosis with sodium bicarbonate. A clearly written protocol sheet is very important. Have cold sterile saline available for wound irrigation, cold IV solution, ice or a cooling blanket, and equipment for cold gastric and rectal lavage. Since succinylcholine and halothane trigger malignant hyperthermia, replace the anesthesia machine with another one, if available. If another anesthesia machine is unavailable, change its circuits and carbon dioxide absorbent. Have a variety of Vacutainer blood vials ready. A warming blanket is contraindicated in malignant hyperthermia.

82. A: The first step in educating a patient about disease management is to assess the patient's knowledge level regarding the disease and his or her general health literacy so that information can be presented in an individualized and culturally appropriate manner. Education should include the purpose of any treatments (such as medications) and any lifestyle changes (such as smoking cessation or diet changes) that may be recommended as well as any resources that are available. It is important to reinforce teaching and allow time for questioning and talk-back and return demonstrations.

83. A: Unscrubbed personnel should not walk between sterile fields. Unscrubbed personnel should keep a safe distance from sterile fields, and should face sterile fields. A mask does not prevent unscrubbed personnel from contaminating a sterile field.

84. A: In an active shooter situation, staff members have very little time to decide on a course of action. The normal response to a fearful situation is the three Fs (i.e., freeze, flight, fight), but staff members need to be retrained to run if they are in imminent danger, hide if they possibly can to avoid the shooter, and fight if they have to protect themselves or others. Fighting most often means throwing whatever is available at the shooter or tackling the shooter. Whenever possible, the staff should call 9-1-1 or yell out warnings to other staff members.

85. B: *Disinfection* is the process that kills pathogenic microorganisms through the application of a chemical germicide, with the exception of bacterial spores. Disinfection does not afford the same level of safety as sterilization. *Purification* means eliminating some unwanted contaminants, such as chlorine or lead. *Fumigation* is gas spray or bombs that eliminate pests, such as bed bugs.

86. A: Efficient turn-over of Operating Rooms between cases is a cost-saving technique. Skipping breaks is not cost-efficient. Perioperative personnel work in a high stress environment and benefit from rest periods. Scratched laser glasses could allow laser beams to damage the eyes. Sterile NSS, once poured, is contaminated.

87. D: While patient safety is of primary concern, the ANA recommends programs that allow for alternatives to disciplinary action; however, the procedures established by the state board of nursing for dealing with impaired nurses, both from substance abuse and psychiatric disorders, must be followed. Some states have adopted the alternative to disciplinary model that allows the nurse to take steps to resolve the problem and return to nursing while other states take more punitive steps. However, in all cases, the problem must be immediately reported and the nurse removed from active duty while impaired.

88. D: National Pressure Injury Advisory Panel (formerly the National Pressure Ulcer Advisory Panel) staging is described as follows:

- 1: Skin is intact; there is localized nonblanchable erythema or blanchable erythema with changes in sensation, temperature, or firmness.
- 2: Partial-thickness skin loss, dermis is exposed, wound bed is viable (pink/red, moist) or intact or ruptured blisters. The adipose tissue and underlying tissues are not exposed.
- 3: Full-thickness skin loss, and adipose tissue and epibole are visible, but underlying tissues (i.e., muscle, tendons, ligaments, cartilage, and bone) are not exposed. Tunneling and undermining may be present.
- 4: Full-thickness loss with underlying tissues exposed or directly palpable. Slough/Eschar may be visible. Epibole, undermining, and tunneling are often present.
- Unstageable: Wound is covered with eschar/slough and unable to stage.

89. A: Introducing a nerve block dose of local medication into the bloodstream can lead to toxicity and a possible cardiac arrest. This can happen during a Bier block if the tourniquet is deflated too quickly.

90. B: When taking telephone orders, the nurse must read back the orders to the physician to ensure that the orders have been properly understood and transcribed. The orders should be read back exactly as written rather than repeated back after the order is given because the nurse may write the order down incorrectly even after repeating it correctly. Asking a second nurse to listen to the order is ineffective as the nurse taking or making the call is responsible for accuracy. For privacy reasons, orders are not generally recorded, and a recording would not ensure accuracy. The physician should only be asked to repeat an order if necessary, for clarification.

91. B: The Veress needle is the portal for inserting CO_2 gas into the patient's abdomen in the closed technique of pneumoperitoneum. The Veress needle has a retractable cutting sheath, which the surgeon inserts through a small supraumbilical incision into the peritoneal cavity. CO_2 tubing attaches to the Veress needle for insufflation.

92. D: While a computerized communication system facilitates hand-off communication by allowing easy access to documents and information, this system is not essential. Nurses must use clear, concise communication techniques, including only approved abbreviations. Procedures for hand-offs should be standardized, including the method of reporting and report forms used. Forms should include all basic information about the procedure, duration, and any complications or unexpected events. Hand-off reports should remain patient-centered, focusing on diagnoses, interventions, and expected outcomes.

93. C: The perioperative nurse should anticipate positioning equipment needed for all patients. The nurse should consider the type of surgery, duration, and use of other equipment to determine the need for special positioning equipment or positioning modifications. For example, obese patients may require lateral transfer devices, beds that can elevate to 30° and/or heavy-duty procedure beds and may be too heavy for standard foam positioning materials. Procedures longer than 3 hours increase the risk of intraoperative pressure injuries.

94. A: Sterile wrappers must be opened in the same manner each time, beginning with the distal (top) flap folded away from the person, then the side flaps, and last the proximal or bottom flap. The edges of the wrappers (usually 1 inch) are considered contaminated. When removing items from the wrapper, the scrub nurse should lift the items straight up and avoid touching the wrapper. The sterile field extends only to the edge of a table.

95. C: The GI surgery patient should *avoid* carbonated beverages for three to four weeks to prevent painful gas bloating.

96. A: When a unique instrument is contaminated during surgery, the circulating nurse dons gloves, retrieves the instrument, sanitizes it, flash sterilizes it, and returns it to the scrub nurse as quickly as possible. The circulating nurse wears gloves for protection against any blood-borne pathogens that may be on the instrument. Sanitizing the instrument removes visible debris only. A sterile towel is unnecessary for picking up a contaminated instrument. Flash sterilization is faster than sending the instrument to CSS. Alcohol and formaldehyde soaks are unacceptable sterilizing techniques.

97. D: Because warfarin has a slow onset of action, unfractionated heparin cannot be stopped abruptly when transitioning to warfarin. Overlapping therapy is usually given for 4–5 days until the patient's INR reaches a therapeutic level of between 2 and 3. If the INR is less than 2, the patient is at risk for a thromboembolic event, but if the INR is greater than 3, the patient is at risk for hemorrhage. The INR must be checked daily until it stabilizes.

98. C: Assess the patient's skin prior to placement of the dispersive electrode. Scar tissue, excessive adipose tissue, metal prosthetic implants, bony prominences, pacemakers, and automatic cardiac defibrillators require special placement of the dispersive electrode.

99. B: *Bariatric surgery* is another term for a weight reduction procedure, such as gastric bypass (stomach stapling). Bariatric patients are morbidly obese, usually 40 kg above their normal weight, or have a BMI above 40. Their health, mobility, environmental access, and socialization have degraded, due to their size.

100. A: Rolled towels and sheets should not be used to reduce pressure and may negate pressure-reducing function of other overlays or pads if placed beneath them. The appropriate pressure-reducing material depends on the patient's weight, position, and duration of surgery. Viscoelastic and gel overlays provide good support for many patients. Thick dense foam compresses less easily and may provide more support than thinner or less dense foam. Obese patients may need special pressure reducing materials. Pressure on the skin should be maintained at ≤ 32 mmHg.

101. A: Place wet towels around the incision site when using a laser. The use of nonreflective instruments prevents the laser beam from reflecting onto unintended areas and possibly causing burns. The laser setting should be on "standby" when not in use.

102. D: Semi critical items include those that come in contact with mucous membranes and nonintact skin, including anesthesia equipment, respiratory equipment, and scopes. Critical items are those that come in contact with sterile tissue and/or the vascular system, including surgical instruments, needles, and angiocatheters. Noncritical items are those that come in contact with intact skin only and have no contact with mucous membranes, including blood pressure cuffs, urinals, bedpans, and assistive devices. Noncritical items include both those items that come in contact with the patient and environmental surfaces.

103. A: Any time the operating table position changes, the scrub nurse should adjust the Mayo stand to an appropriate height, taking care not to injure the patient. Never allow the Mayo stand to contact the patient. If a step stool improves the view of the surgical field, request one.

104. C: The type of glove used by the surgical technologist determines her latex exposure level. If she noticed a latex reaction, such as rash after removal of the gloves, it could indicate a potentially lethal latex allergy. Food allergies may also be indicative of the potential for latex allergies. Allergies to bananas, avocados, kiwis, and chestnuts are particularly predictive of a latex allergy. Her area of specialization is unimportant for her safety, so asking her about it would just serve as an icebreaker.

105. C: Anxiety produces *slight* hypertension, increased pulse, and increased respiratory rates and is normal before any stressful event, such as surgery. Hypertension, COPD, and heart disease should appear in the Medical History section of the patient's *Preassessment Information Sheet.*

106. D: Semi-restricted areas include sterile and clean supply storage, work areas to store and process instruments and supplies, corridors leading to operating rooms, and scrub sinks. Only authorized personnel and patients are allowed in this area. Staff must wear surgical attire and cover facial hair. Unrestricted areas are those outside the doors to the surgical suite. Restricted areas include operating and procedure rooms and the clean core area. Staff must wear surgical attire and hair covering.

107. A: A member of the surgical team who contaminates a glove must step away from the sterile field, wait for the circulating nurse to remove the contaminated glove, and finally re-glove.

108. B: The single lumen, rubber or silicone, Penrose drain is the most common *passive* drain. The Jackson-Pratt and Hemovac are *active* drains, in which the reservoir collapses to create negative pressure, directing the drainage into the reservoir. *Sump drains* are double-lumened and may attach to an external suction machine.

109. B: Pressing the staple firmly against the incision can cause unnecessary trauma. A better technique is to "kiss" the skin gently with the stapler when applying skin staples. Place staples ¼ inch apart.

110. B: *Cutting-point* needles have a razor-sharp tip for easily penetrating tough tissues, such as skin or tendon. *Taper-point* needles are appropriate for soft tissue, such as intestine or peritoneum. Blunt-tip needles are suitable for friable tissue, such as liver or kidney. "Saber-tip" is a misnomer.

111. C: Occupational hazards in the nurse's workplace include: Needle sticks; slips and falls; head injuries; chemical, radiation, and anesthetic gas exposures; and back injuries. Occupational hazards lead many nurses to leave their profession. Nurses in the OR wear personal protective equipment (PPE) when exposed to infectious materials. Depending on the facility, most nurses have choices regarding their preferred hours of work. There are difficult people in every profession. Disagreeable surgeons are not a recognized reason for nurses leaving their profession.

112. A: Evidence-based practice is the systematic, meticulous process used to identify an issue, to gather and assess the best evidence to draft and employ a practice change and to evaluate the process.

113. B: Firstly, establish the requirements for the new drape materials. Secondly, contact multiple manufacturers and have their representatives set up product demonstrations. Thirdly, compare costs and quality from one manufacturer to the next, including thickness of the drape material and fire-resistance. Evaluate single drapes vs. combination packages with cost comparisons. Other considerations include ease of use, staff opinions of sample materials, and environmental impact from disposal.

114. C: The *Sellick maneuver* involves pressing on the patient's cricoid cartilage with the index finger, or thumb and forefinger. The Sellick maneuver provides better visualization of the tracheal lumen and occludes the esophagus to prevent regurgitation.

115. B: TPR, skin appearance, and level of consciousness are parts of the physical assessment, not the psychosocial assessment. Psychosocial assessment means estimating the patient's: Capacity to understand the surgical procedure; coping ability; comprehension and inclination to learn; anxiety level regarding the procedure and outcome; knowledge of perioperative practices; and cultural or spiritual beliefs, as they relate to the procedure.

116. C: *First and foremost,* remove the drapes to rescue the patient from the burning materials. Next, announce over the intercom system, "Code Red" and the location of fire. Turn off all room gases. Contain the fire. Extinguish it with water or saline from the back table, or with the halon fire extinguisher. When the fire is out, announce, "Code Red, all clear."

117. D: Forced air warming in which a special blanket or garment provides warm air blowing over the skin is a safe and widely used method of preventing hypothermia and may maintain temperature even if only 50% of the body is covered. Circulating-water garments and energy transfer pads that also circulate warm water may also be used. Warming IV fluids is not a skin surface warming method but is effective only with large volumes (more than 2 L/h for adults). If other methods are not feasible, then increasing the ambient temperature to more than 73.4 °F (23 °C) may help reduce heat loss.

118. B: Steam sterilization is the oldest, safest, cheapest, and best understood method. Ethylene oxide is highly explosive, carcinogenic, toxic, and flammable. Dry heat takes two hours, so it is only appropriate for materials that cannot tolerate other methods of sterilization, such as powders, grease, anhydrous oils, and some glassware. Low-temperature hydrogen peroxide plasma is replacing ethylene oxide, but *Geobacillus stearothermophilus* spores may survive peroxidation.

119. B: In the open gloving technique, there is a greater chance of contamination. Closed gloving, gloving by another scrub personnel, and double gloving are the safer gloving techniques.

120. A: The grass allergy is irrelevant to the surgical procedure, unless it is performed in the field. Paralysis is important for positioning and for transferring the patient. The history and location of implants are relevant when using electrocoagulation. The fact that the patient's brother (or any direct family member) had a "bad reaction to anesthesia" must be communicated to the OR nurse, and then to the surgeon, and investigated prior to surgery. The reaction being referred to may have been malignant hyperthermia, in which case it is a genetic predisposition, and tests may need to be run prior to initiating surgery.

121. C: The OR supervisor must have a blend of management, clinical, interpersonal, technological, and financial expertise. Central Sterilization techniques expertise is not a minimum qualification for an OR supervisor.

122. B: Yes/No questions should be avoided in interviews. Questioning techniques include:

- Ask information questions with "who," "what," "where," "when," and "how," but avoid questions with "why" if possible:
    - Instead of "Why do you continue to eat sugar?" ask, "What sugar substitutes have you tried?"
- Ask brief clarifying questions: "How long were you in the hospital?"
- Provide a list of options: "Is your headache throbbing, stabbing, or dull?
- Rephrase/reflect to encourage clarification:
    - Patient: "My aunt had this same surgery and died a month later."
    - Nurse: "You're afraid you might die from this surgery?"

123. A: Although all of these forms contain important information, the patient's consent is the only one of the four reviewed for verification of the procedure.

124. B: The Joint Commission, the Association of periOperative Registered Nurses (AORN), and the World Health Organization (WHO) all recommend against wearing artificial nails. Chipped or broken artificial nails harbor significantly more microorganisms. *Well-maintained* nail polish does not increase the microorganism count; therefore, no action is necessary.

125. B:

- Class I: Clean wounds (risk < 2%) do not enter an area of the body that is usually colonized by normal flora.
- Class II: Clean-contaminated wounds (risk < 10%) enter into colonized parts of the body, such as the respiratory or urinary tract.
- Class III: Contaminated wounds (risk 20%) have obvious inflammation but no purulent discharge. They may involve spillage of the gastrointestinal tract, penetrating wounds (<4 hours), and/or substantial break in aseptic technique.
- Class IV: Dirty-infected wounds (risk 40%) show obvious inflammation and purulent discharge. There may be perforation of viscera prior to surgery and/or penetrating wounds (>4 hours).

126. B: To prevent injury during surgery, move a patient into the lithotomy position by lifting the patient's legs carefully, *slowly and in unison* to prevent injury to the sacroiliac joint. Legs should then be secured in leg supports to prevent movement during surgery. Moving the legs one at a time may cause injury to the patient.

127. C: Schedule patients with airborne-transmitted diseases, such as tuberculosis (TB), to have surgery when personnel and patients are at a minimum (last case of the day).

128. A: Phlebothrombosis may result if blood flow to the patient's legs is obstructed. Shearing results from moving the patient improperly. Air embolism is an air bubble floating in the circulatory system. Bronchospasm may occur upon extubation, but is not a result of faulty positioning.

129. C: If a patient is showing signs of an adverse reaction to local anesthetic the nurse should inform the surgeon of the signs and symptoms the patient is experiencing. They should establish and maintain an airway and administer oxygen, and give sedation as ordered by the surgeon. Call the anesthesiologist for assistance, if necessary. Ensure the crash cart (resuscitation equipment) is in the room. Narcan is a drug used to counter the action of narcotics, not local anesthetics.

130. C: The surgical patient who ingested food or liquid within 8 hours of surgery requires special precautions to prevent potentially fatal aspiration of gastric contents while under anesthesia. Standing by, the perioperative nurse should have a nasogastric tube, an emesis basin, a suction catheter with a soft tip, and a clean towel. Sterilization of this towel is unnecessary. The perioperative nurse must also be prepared to use the Sellick maneuver, which occludes the esophagus in an intubated patient and helps prevent aspiration.

131. C: Once the scrub nurse wears the gown, its cuffs, neckline, shoulder, and axillae are not sterile. The area below the waist and the back are not sterile. Sterile areas include the top edge of the cuffs to two inches above the elbow, and the front of the gown, from the chest to the level of the sterile field.

132. B: The circulating nurse and the scrub nurse that perform the counts should sign the Perioperative Report. If a scrub technician is utilized instead of a scrub nurse, then only the circulating nurse would sign the report since the scrub technician cannot be a part of the documentation process. The documentation should identify all individuals who were part of the sponge counting process.

133. B: Obesity increases the patient's risk of infection, due to the decreased blood supply in adipose tissue. Radiation therapy patients are immunocompromised and more prone to infection. The administration of immunosuppressants post-operatively, commonly after transplants to prevent rejection, also increases a patient's risk of infection. Previous joint replacement should not increase the risk of infection for a patient's future surgeries.

134. B: Category II. The Payne–Martin Classification for Skin Tears is categorized as follows:

Category	Skin Loss	Description
I	Skin tear without tissue loss	Linear: Full-thickness wound (incisional appearance) or partial-thickness wound with a flap. Flap: Partial-thickness wound with a flap that can cover the wound with ≤ 1 mm of dermis exposed. The epidermis and dermis are separated.
II	Skin tear with partial tissue loss	Scant tissue loss: Partial-thickness injury and ≤25% of the epidermal flap is lost. Moderate–large tissue loss: Partial-thickness injury with >25% of the epidermal flap is lost.
III	Skin tear with complete tissue loss	Open area with no epidermal flap.

135. B: An improperly placed, heavy, third trimester uterus pressurizes the vena cava and aorta, resulting in hypotension. Put a padded wedge under her right side to tilt her uterus laterally and alleviate pressure on the major vessels. Raising the patient's legs prevents venous pooling in her lower extremities, but does not relieve uterine pressure on her heart. A small pillow under her waist may improve her comfort in the supine position, but does not decrease the uterine burden. Sequential compression stockings prevent blood from pooling in the legs, but have no effect on the pressure the uterus applies to the major blood vessels of the heart.

136. C: Kittners, lap pads, RAY-TEC® sponges, peanuts, tonsil sponges and cottonoid patties are all countable items. Thrombin-soaked gelatin sponges are not countable, since the body absorbs them, and they control bleeding.

137. D: Thrombin customarily comes from dried beef blood. Thrombin combines with fibrinogen to accelerate the coagulation process, and is useful for controlling capillary bleeding. Thrombin is dispensed as a white powder, which the scrub nurse mixes with sterile water or saline, and uses in conjunction with a gelatin sponge. Thrombin retains its potency for about three hours, but works best if used shortly after mixing. Thrombin is for *topical use only, never for injection*. Bovine-derived thrombin can lead to an autoimmune response, resulting in a severe bleeding complication.

138. B: Second-degree burn. Degrees of injury associated with burns are detailed below:

Degree	Depth/Extent	Description
First	Superficial, epidermis only	Mild pain, erythema, slight edema, no blistering. Heals within 3–7 days.
Second	Through epidermis and into dermis	Moderate to severe pain, erythema, large watery blisters, edema. Heals within 2–3 weeks.
Third	Through the epidermis, dermis, and into underlying tissues	Pain levels vary because surrounding tissue may have first- or second-degree burns, but patients may have little pain in third-degree burns if nerve endings are destroyed. Tissues may appear white, brown, or black. Skin grafting may be necessary.

139. A: Ophthalmic instruments are very delicate. Eye instruments must be hand-washed and their tips carefully examined *before use* for burrs. They should not be sent to CSS for processing or washed mechanically due to their delicate nature.

140. A: Reattach her urinary catheter bag to a lower section of the cart to permit gravity drainage. If the scrub nurse places the drainage bag on the patient's abdomen, the urine drains back into her bladder, increasing her discomfort and chances of a urinary tract infection. Clamping the catheter and detaching it from the drainage tubing during transport would be time-consuming. Since it is imperative to move the patient to the Post Anesthesia Care Unit (PACU) as quickly as possible, the best choice is to hang her bag on a lower section of the cart.

141. B: Surgical preps begin at the incision site and moves outward in a spiral motion to the periphery. Most prep solutions require a 20-minute wait to ensure optimal killing of surface microorganisms.

142. C: In this scenario, the best response is to remove the sterile 3" x3" gauze pads from the back table to eliminate their possible use in the current surgery. *Never* use a sponge on a sponge stick that does not have a radiopaque strip, in case it is retained and the patient must be reopened.

143. B: Grade II radiation burn. The grades of radiation injury/burns are described below:

Grade	Description
Grade I	Slight inflammation and edema. Vessels dilate and capillaries are more permeable, causing erythema. The patient may have itching, burning, or pain.
Grade II	Dry, itchy, scaly skin with partial sloughing of the epidermis. Itching, burning, and pain increase.
Grade III	Moist, blistering skin with loss of epidermal tissue, resulting in serous drainage. Exposed nerves cause increased pain.
Grade IV	Permanent hair loss, tissue atrophy, pigment changes, and ulcerations.

144. D: Surgical patients who are most likely to contract MRSA include: High-risk patients with underlying diseases; those with prolonged hospitalizations; patients from Intensive Care Units; patients who have had previous antimicrobial therapy; and those who were exposed to other MRSA patients.

145. A: The nurse who is monitoring a sedated patient should have *no other responsibilities*. A second perioperative nurse should circulate, and a third nurse should "scrub in" to assist the surgeon.

146. C: A hospital-grade disinfectant that is approved by the EPA is appropriate for use in the OR *prior* to the first case of the day. Alcohol and high-level disinfectants used for instruments are inappropriate for use as cleansers in the OR because they are flammable. Formalin is a specimen preservative, but as a proven carcinogen, it is unsuitable as a cleanser. If the surgeon used cadaverous transplant material, or the patient had rapid-onset dementia, or the family history is suspicious for prion diseases, soak the instruments after surgery in a covered pan of 1N sodium hydroxide (NaOH) for 60 minutes, steam autoclave for 30 minutes at 121 °C, AND follow up with routine sterilization. Check the CDC and WHO Web sites for the latest CJD decontamination techniques.

147. B: Increasing power on the ultrasonic scalpel increases the cutting speed but decreases its coagulation capability. An ultrasonic scalpel vibrates at 55,000 times per second, allowing it to cut and coagulate simultaneously at temperatures lower than electrosurgery. The denatured protein creates a sticky coagulant.

148. D: One of the many things that should be checked during the head-to-toe assessment is the neurovascular area. Assessing peripheral pulses is one method to do this.

149. C: The Nurse's Five Rights of Delegation include the right task, right circumstances, right person, right communication, and right supervision. Right diagnosis and status are not part of the Five Rights of Delegation.

150. B: The patient who receives local anesthetic may have a *toxic reaction* from rapid absorption by the circulatory system. Signs and symptoms of a toxic reaction (from mild to severe) are restlessness, dizziness, visual and auditory disturbances, tremors, convulsions, unconsciousness, apnea, and cardiac arrest.

151. B: The most common cause of delayed wound healing is SSI.

Superficial incisional:

- ≤30 days
- Purulent discharge, organisms isolated, signs of infection, and wound opened or physician diagnosis

Deep incisional:

- ≤ 30 days if there is no implant (1 year with implant)
- Purulent discharge, signs of infections, and incision dehiscence or deliberately opened
- Abscess or other evidence of infection or physician diagnosis

Organ space:

- ≤30 days of surgery if there is no implant (1 year with implant) and the infection appears related
- Infection of any part of body (organs, tissues) manipulated during surgery
- Purulent discharge evident from drain to organ/space, organisms isolated from fluids or tissue in organ space, abscess in area, or diagnosis by physician

152. A: During laser surgery, the smoke evacuation suction tube should be held 1 inch, or as close as possible, from the tissue interaction site to contain the plume (smoke, particles). The type of smoke evacuation system used depends on the laser and the amount of plume generated. The tubing used for the system should be smooth on the interior to prevent excess noise. Filters on the suctioning equipment should be changed according to manufacturer's directions. Surgical smoke should also be suctioned during endoscopic procedures.

153. A: The scrub nurse must label all medications on the sterile field with either pre-printed labels or plain sterile labels with a sterile marker. The use of different containers helps identify the medication from a distance, but the container must have the name of the drug printed on it as a fail-safe. Permanent markers should not be a first- or second-line use for medication identification.

154. B: TEE monitoring is an invasive tool that is the best way to monitor myocardial ischemia. It can also be useful in cardiac valve surgeries, examining the problems before and the effectiveness of the repair after.

155. A: A metal implant in a patient's right hip means that the perioperative nurse must avoid putting the metal implant in the circuit path between the active electrode and the dispersive electrode pad. An extra-large dispersive pad is not necessary.

156. B: A clean wound (Class I) means the patient's GI, respiratory, or GU tract are intact (not entered). A clean contaminated wound (Class II) means the surgeon entered the patient's GI, respiratory, or GU tract by controlled means. A contaminated wound (Class III) is grossly (visibly) contaminated with a foreign substance, but there is no sign of infection. A dirty or infected wound (Class IV) means the surgical site contains infected or dead (necrotic) tissue.

157. C: During intubation, the perioperative nurse can: Pull *outwardly* on the corner of the patient's mouth to enhance visualization of the vocal chords; hold the endotracheal tube for easy access by the anesthetist; apply pressure (the Sellick maneuver) to the *cricoid cartilage* to enhance chord exposure: and provide a 10 mL syringe for inflation of the endotracheal tube cuff.

158. C: To activate the fire extinguisher, the nurse must pull the extinguisher's pin, aim the nozzle, squeeze the handle, and then sweep the stream at the base of the fire. Starting the spray at the top of the fire and then sweeping down is not the most effective use of the extinguisher.

159. A: Air embolism is a potential complication of intercostal nerve blocks.

160. D: The Association of periOperative Registered Nurses (AORN) provides educational resources and continuing education courses and conferences. AORN also develops evidence-based guidelines for perioperative practice (such as medication safety, manual high-level disinfection, team communication, and safe patient handling and movement), supports research regarding perioperative nursing, and advocates for public policies and legislature that support the profession. AORN also offers certification programs such as certified perioperative nurse credentialing through the Competency and Credentialing Institute.

161. C: *Shearing injuries* result when the tissue below the skin moves but the skin remains stationary. Shearing may be the consequence of pulling a patient instead of lifting him. The patient's subcutaneous capillaries tear, causing tissue ischemia, which may progress to a pressure injury. An inadequately padded bony prominence may also lead to a tissue injury after more than 20 minutes of direct weight-bearing, but this is an example of a *pressure injury* that is not secondary to shearing.

162. D: Patients with spinal cord injuries at or above T6 are at risk for autonomic dysreflexia, which results in a sudden, dramatic increase in BP. The patient is immediately seated in high Fowler's position to take advantage of postural hypotension, and the clothes are loosened because anything that puts pressure on the skin can trigger the reaction. If these measures are ineffective, bladder function (e.g., distention, blocked catheter) is assessed next; however, the Credé maneuver must be avoided. Then, bowel function is assessed with manual examination using a topical anesthetic, such as lidocaine, before beginning, in order to avoid further triggering. If the BP remains high, antihypertensives are indicated.

163. A: Laparoscopy requires specialized surgical training and can usually only be used for elective surgery, not emergencies. However, it offers the patient many advantages, including: Decreased blood loss; reduced infection risk; increased return of GI function; diminished chance of small bowel obstruction; lowered risk of incisional hernia; and reduced postoperative pain.

164. A: Use the "time out" prior to starting the surgical procedure to verify the patient's identify, ensure the correct procedure is on record and verbally understood, the right site is marked, and all surgical implants are readily available (if applicable). It also ensures that the surgical team is on the same page and prepared for surgery. The surgical "time out" is a standardized safety protocol that is not related to staff breaks. Surgical staff only take breaks when relieved by other qualified staff members.

165. B: When returning a patient to the supine position from the lithotomy position, remove her feet from the stirrups, extend her legs completely to avoid abduction of the hips, close them, and then slowly lower them. Bend at the knees rather than the hips/back to prevent back injury. Severe hypotension can result from lowering the legs too quickly, since 500 mL to 800 mL of blood diverts from the viscera to the lower extremities.

166. B: Once the drape slides off the surgical area, it becomes contaminated. The student nurse must remove the contaminated drape, discard it, and obtain a sterile replacement. Placing the contaminated drape on the sterile back table would contaminate the back table. Reprepping the surgical site is unnecessary; the draping material was originally sterile and only became contaminated when it shifted to the unprepped area.

167. D: Arteriovenous fistula patients are at risk for hemorrhage at the fistula site. This risk does not dissipate after surgery. These patients are at risk for a life-threatening hemorrhage even years after the procedure if the fistula develops an aneurysm.

168. B: Gender politics can be difficult to maneuver. If a patient's medical record identifies the patient as male, he has not legally transitioned to female, and one cannot assume that a patient is transgender simply by appearances because some patients identify as nonbinary. The best solution when encountering a patient whose gender orientation is not clear is to ask the patient what pronouns the patient uses. If the patient identifies as she/her and by a different name (such as Roberta), then the patient's care plan should reflect that choice, and the patient should be referred to accordingly.

169. C: Before applying alcohol in an alcohol-based surgical hand scrub, the person should wash the hands and forearms with nonantimicrobial soap and dry thoroughly. The alcohol-based product should be used according to manufacturer's directions. After application of the alcohol-based product, the skin should be thoroughly air dried before gloves are applied. When doing an antimicrobial scrub, the hands and forearms should be washed according to manufacturer's directions, usually for 2-6 minutes.

170. C: Carbon dioxide (CO_2) lasers *can* damage the *cornea*. Water in the surface cells of the cornea absorbs the CO_2 laser's beam, resulting in an immediate, painful burn. Argon and Nd:YAG lasers can damage the *retina.* The lens of the eye refocuses the beam of the Argon and Nd:YAG laser and can damage the retina with no accompanying pain. Eye protection is very important during *any* procedure in which laser therapy is used, regardless of the gas. Even low levels of laser radiation can lead to permanent eye injury.

171. A: The Richardson, Army-Navy and Deaver are all retractors. The Allis, Babcock and Kocher are grasping clamps. The towel clip and sponge forceps are also grasping clamps. Metzenbaum, Mayo and Castroviejo are types of scissors.

172. C: Adjustable gastric bands to have a possible complication of tissue erosion if the band slips. Incisional hernia formation, anastomosis leakage, and anastomotic stricture are complications specific to gastric bypass procedures.

173. A: Malignant hyperthermia is a life-threatening condition triggered in those with the genetic susceptibility by inhalational anesthetics, including halothane, isoflurane, enflurane, sevoflurane, desflurane, and succinylcholine, as well as other medications (epinephrine, digitalis) and stress. Nitrous oxide, barbiturates, propofol, opioids, ketamine, etomidate, nondepolarizing muscle relaxants, and local and regional anesthetics do not trigger malignant hyperthermia. Malignant hyperthermia results in increased cytoplasmic calcium, hypermetabolism, and cell leakage of potassium, myoglobin, and creatine phosphokinase (damaging cells).

174. C: Nitrous oxide is "laughing gas", a sweet-smelling, analgesic gas that rapidly produces mild euphoria and relaxation. It is a *supplement,* used in combination with stronger inhaled anesthetics to improve their action. Nitrous oxide is not a stand-alone anesthetic.

175. B: The proper procedure for attaching a blade to a scalpel handle is to use the needle holder to attach and remove blades to prevent injuries. Never touch the blade, or use the packaging to apply the blade to the handle. Toothed forceps would not create a firm grip on the blade.

176. B: Mass casualty events result in large numbers of patients in need of care, such as with a pandemic, but the infrastructure remains generally intact, at least in the early stages. Mass effect events, however—which include most types of natural disasters, such as hurricanes, earthquakes, floods, and tornadoes—often result in infrastructure disruption. For example, power may be out, communication may be severed, and roads may be impassable. Emergency preparedness plans must take into account the possible results of mass effect events as well as mass casualty events.

177. C: The insufflation of CO_2 begins at a rate of 1 to 2 L/min, with a *maximum pressure level of 15 mmHg*. Higher pressures could result in CO_2 diffusion into the bloodstream, with ensuing respiratory acidosis, bradycardia, blood pressure changes, and possibly lethal gas embolism.

178. C: Once a nurse touches the faucet with her hand, the hand is contaminated. The appropriate action is to start the scrub over from the beginning, using a new scrub sponge or brush. Proceeding into the OR with a contaminated hand, rinsing for an extra minute, or double-gloving are unacceptable, high-risk actions. The only safe choice is to begin again.

179. B: At least two people are necessary to transfer the patient from the stretcher to the operating table. Lock the wheels of the stretcher *and* operating table prior to moving the patient. Never assume the cleaner remembered to lock the operating table after disinfecting it; ensure the OR table will not roll. The stretcher should be the *same* level as the operating table prior to transferring the patient, not higher.

180. C: Methyl methacrylate is an acrylic, cement-type compound used in some orthopedic and neurosurgery cases. The nurse removes his/her contact lenses to prevent eye damage from penetrating vapors. Wear a face shield and double gloves. Mix the chemicals under a fume hood or suction evacuation bowl *without* electronic equipment. Ensure there are no sparks or open flames, as the liquid component is highly flammable. Pour the liquid (PMMA) into the powder, to minimize aerosolization. Polymerization will form the compound into a durable plastic.

181. C: Steam sterilization may damage some plastics, melt some powders, and dilute some oils. Steam is readily available and leaves no toxic residue. Steam is economical and fast. Steam is appropriate for most surgical instruments and in-house packaging materials.

182. D: Performance improvement techniques encompass improvements in quality and effectiveness, based on moral and economical perspectives.

183. D: Indications of transurethral resection syndrome associated with intra- or extravasation of irrigation fluids include bradycardia, hypotension, chest pain, and hyponatremia. Intravasation occurs when irrigating fluid enters the bloodstream through cut or injured vessels, and extravasation occurs when fluid diffuses from a blood vessel into the surrounding tissue, resulting in edema. Monitoring for fluid deficits is important for quickly identifying intravasation.

184. A: Blunt suture-tip needles provide safer alternatives for prevention of percutaneous injuries in the OR. They are appropriate for use on internal tissue, not for use on skin closure. Blunt suture-tip needles come in a range of bluntness in several gauges.

185. B: If heat is lost when air currents move across the skin, such as from an air conditioning vent, this type of heat loss is convective. If the air is cooler than the body, then radiant heat loss occurs as heat transfers to the environment. With conductive heat loss, heat transfers through direct contact from a warmer person/object to a cooler one. With evaporative heat loss, water (perspiration) converts to a gas, resulting in cooling.

186. C: Electric clipping is the preferred method for removing hair from a surgical site. A razor blade may nick the area and increase the chances of infection. Hot wax pulls the hair and may result in inflammation of the area.

187. A: The Universal Protocol for prevention of wrong site, wrong procedure, or wrong person surgeries has three steps:

1. *Preoperative verification process,* which assures that all relevant test results and documents are available before the procedure begins, have been reviewed, and are consistent with the planned procedure.
2. *Marking of the operative site* with a permanent marker, after verifying the location and procedure with the patient, family member or other responsible party is extremely important. This mark must remain visible after the patient's prep and draping for surgery.
3. Taking a "time out" in the OR immediately prior to starting the surgical procedure, to verify the correct identity of the patient, the exact site of the proposed incision, the right scheduled procedure, and the availability of implants, if applicable.

188. B: Freshly applied fingernail polish does not pose increased safety risk and can be worn, but chipped nail polish or nail polish worn for at least 4 days increases risk of bacterial contamination. Nails should be kept short and clean. Artificial nails prevent adequate hand cleaning and may harbor gram-negative microorganisms and fungi. Rings may also harbor bacteria and should be removed. Necklaces may contaminate the surgical field and surgical attire if not properly confined, so for safety reasons they should be removed.

189. A: The circulating nurse is responsible for recording incision time, end of surgery time and anesthesia induction time. The temperature of the room is not recorded on the OR record.

190. B: Bladder perforation can occur during a transurethral prostatectomy because of overinflation of the bladder with irrigant or surgical instrumentation. An early indication is a decrease in return flow of bladder irrigant, so the nurse should monitor the irrigation fluids carefully. As fluid flows into the abdomen through the perforation, the abdomen becomes rigid and swollen, and the patient may complain of abdominal pain and experience nausea and vomiting. The patient may become hypotensive and later hypertensive.

191. D: Deep vein thrombosis is a risk factor for total knee arthroplasty because of the interruption of blood flow during the procedure and immobility during and after the procedure. In some cases, vessels may be damaged by the surgical procedure and veins may be compressed. Additionally, the body naturally increases the ability of the blood to clot as a protective mechanism in response to surgery. Signs and symptoms include pain, edema, and erythema. Preexisting conditions, such as obesity, varicose veins, and prolonged immobility, increase risk.

192. C: Among many others, gastroesophageal reflux disease, also known as GERD, is an associated disease with morbid obesity. This is significant to surgical procedures because the patient's gag reflex is unprotected when given anesthesia and the patient may aspirate. Providing cricoid pressure during induction is often requested for this purpose.

193. D: Pulmonary edema is a contraindication to pneumatic compression therapy because the increased venous return may exacerbate the pulmonary edema. Other contraindications include severe peripheral arterial disease (ankle-brachial index test <0.6, systolic ankle pressure <60 mmHg, to pressure <320 mmHg), severe arteriosclerosis, heart failure (New York Heart Association Functional Classification IV), hypoproteinemia, skin infection or a recent skin graft on the lower extremities, or severe diabetic neuropathy with loss of sensation.

194. C: *Appropriate* eye-wear is necessary for all laser surgeries, even endoscopic. Laser glasses are specific to the type of laser used. Laser precautions include: Place "Danger, Laser Radiation" signs on all entrances to the OR; cover all windows; hang extra laser eye-wear outside the doors, so anyone entering will be protected; place wet gauze pads on the anesthetized patient's eyes; provide protective eye-wear for the conscious patient; and use nonreflective instruments.

195. B: A large percentage of fires in the OR occur in the patient's facial area because of the oxygen-enriched atmosphere. Fires during abdominal surgeries may be due to ignition of the drape material by an active electrode.

196. B: Delirium is characterized by fluctuating signs and symptoms, and this fluctuation helps differentiate delirium from disorders with similar symptoms. Patients may exhibit a sudden change in consciousness with a reduced ability to focus or sustain attention, language and memory disturbances, disorientation, confusion, audiovisual hallucinations, sleep disturbance, and psychomotor activity disorder. The Confusion Assessment Method is used to assess a patient for delirium. Patients may require a sitter for safety. Medications may include trazodone, lorazepam, and haloperidol.

197. B: Shaving the patient in the OR could result in airborne hair contamination of the sterile fields. The Holding Area, where the patient awaits surgery, is the preferred location for the preoperative shave.

198. D: BCIS is characterized by pulmonary hypertension, which can lead to right ventricular dysfunction and hypotension. In severe cases, sudden death may occur. BCIS is associated with the use of bone cement (primarily methyl methacrylate) to secure hip prostheses, with symptoms occurring within minutes. The cause is now believed to be medullary fat embolism caused by the glue sealing and increasing pressure in the femoral canal when the prosthesis is inserted rather than a reaction to the glue itself. Cementless procedures decrease risk.

199. A: The best method of transfer for dirty instruments is in a closed cart, to prevent inadvertent contamination of other hospital areas during transportation. Other methods present opportunities for the instruments to come in contact with the environment.

200. C: The scrub nurse should leave these items on the back table until there is time to open and count them with the circulating nurse. The scrub nurse cannot count these items without the circulating nurse present, and the circulating nurse cannot count these items without the scrub nurse. Both must count together. In this case, the scrub nurse should pass the surgeon the next instrument, then open and count the items with the circulating nurse.

CNOR Practice Test #2

1. A circulating RN is assisting the anesthesia care provider with a general anesthesia induction on a patient with a history of gastroesophageal reflux disease (GERD). The anesthesia care provider asks the nurse to perform cricoid pressure. What is the purpose of cricoid pressure?

a. To keep the patient's neck stable during tube placement.
b. To open the esophagus and allow air to enter the stomach to prevent gastric acid regurgitation.
c. To prevent aspiration of gastric contents while the patient does not have a proper gag reflex.
d. To hide the vocal cords because they are not a needed landmark to intubate.

2. Which of the following IV solutions is contraindicated for a patient in an MH crisis?

a. Lactated Ringer's (LR).
b. Normal saline (NS).
c. Dextrose (D5).
d. Potassium chloride (KCL).

3. A patient is going into respiratory arrest after a 2 mg dose of Versed. Which of the following medications would be the most appropriate to reverse the effects of this medication?

a. Romazicon.
b. Narcan.
c. Benadryl.
d. Epinephrine.

4. In which of the following scenarios would it be acceptable for the scrub nurse to open her sterile gown and gloves on the sterile back table?

a. It is never recommended to do this.
b. When there is a sterile member, such as the scrub nurse she is relieving, to gown and glove her.
c. When there is no other surface available.
d. Once the patient has been draped, but the skin incision has not yet been made.

5. At the conclusion of a stable carotid endarterectomy surgery, after extubation the anesthesia care provider may ask the circulating RN to get a laryngoscope or glidescope. Which of the following provides the best rationale for this request?

a. To emergently reintubate the patient.
b. To check if the vocal cords are responding.
c. To check for bleeding.
d. To properly suction the patient.

6. The circulating RN is unwrapping a sterile endoscope for the sterile scrub tech. Which of the following best describes the technique used when unwrapping a sterile instrument as an unsterile person?

a. Open the top flap away from oneself, then the sides, and then the bottom, being careful not to let the flaps touch each other so the edges do not contaminate each other.
b. Open the top flap away from oneself, then the sides, and then the bottom, securing each flap so they cover the unsterile hand and do not contaminate the sterile field or instrument.
c. The scrub tech should open sterile items because she is already sterile.
d. No real method exists as long as the nurse does not touch the sterile item.

7. The surgeon asks the scrub nurse in the operating room for a fenestrated drape. Which of the following gives the best definition of what a fenestrated drape is?

a. A drape with openings.
b. A folded towel.
c. Any folded drape.
d. An adhesive clear drape.

8. Which of the following is the best method to prevent intraoperative patient burns when using an electrosurgical unit (ESU)?

a. Leave the ESU pencil on the surgical drape in open view between uses.
b. Ensure adequate skin contact of the patient return electrode.
c. Place the patient return electrode over a previous surgical site.
d. Do not use any alcohol-based surgical preps in the operating room.

9. Which of the following are potential complications of a mediastinoscopy?

a. Recurrent laryngeal nerve injury.
b. Pulmonary edema.
c. Cardiac tamponade.
d. Esophageal tears.

10. As the circulating RN caring for a patient receiving a Bier block, which of the following is a very important consideration at the conclusion of the procedure with this type of anesthesia?

a. Once the tourniquet is released, the surgical site will have a large amount of drainage.
b. These patients have a great deal of pain once the tourniquet is released.
c. There are no different concerns with Bier blocks than any other anesthesia.
d. The tourniquet should be released slowly to prevent a bolus of medication into the patient.

11. When performing a skin prep, the circulating nurse must be aware of the body parts that are considered contaminated in relation the surgical site, so she will know how to prep. For an abdominal surgery, what site should be cleaned first?

a. Incision site.
b. Breast.
c. Lower abdomen.
d. Umbilicus.

12. Laryngeal nerve paralysis is a potential complication of which block?

a. Celiac block.
b. Intercostal block.
c. Intraocular block.
d. Brachial plexus.

13. Knowing the intraoperative positioning required for a gastric band placement, which of the following additional pieces of equipment would be necessary?

a. Allen stirrups.
b. Footboard.
c. Shoulder roll.
d. Axillary roll.

14. Who has the responsibility to obtain informed consent?

a. Surgeon.
b. Circulating RN.
c. Primary MD.
d. Preoperative RN.

15. Which of the following best describes the purpose of informed consent?

a. To prevent health information privacy violations.
b. To inform the patient of which physician will be performing the procedure.
c. To explain to the patient the type and purpose of the procedure as well as the risks, benefits, alternatives, and complications associated with it.
d. To alleviate the legal burden of a poor outcome.

16. What is the primary purpose of the surgical skin prep?

a. To sterilize the surgical site.
b. To eliminate skin flora.
c. To reduce skin flora by chemically decontaminating the site.
d. To degrease the skin.

17. The information the nurse must document when a tourniquet is used during surgery includes

a. an assessment of the skin above the tourniquet, and the type of skin protection used under the cuff.
b. the tourniquet's location, cuff pressure, calibration, and times of inflation and deflation.
c. the cuff material and the condition of the opposite limb for comparison.
d. the calibration pressure and the equipment's usage history.

18. Which of the following personnel safety precautions is most appropriate for the scrub nurse for a surgery using a laser?

a. Wearing a mask with a splash shield.
b. Wearing safety goggles with the correct optical density for the laser being used.
c. Wearing a standard surgical mask.
d. Wearing latex-free gloves.

19. A nurse has forgotten the personal password needed to access a patient's EHR and uses the password of a coworker to access the records of the patient to whom the nurse is assigned. This is a(n)

a. permissible use of a password.
b. example of negligence.
c. felony offense.
d. HIPAA violation.

20. Which of the following is a discharge criterion of Phase II but not Phase I of the postanesthesia care unit (PACU)?

a. Airway patency.
b. Pain level.
c. Level of consciousness.
d. Gag reflex.

21. Any healthcare facility that procures and/or stores human tissue for transfer to another facility must do which of the following?

a. Register with the Department of Human Services (DHS) as a tissue bank.
b. Register with the Food & Drug Administration (FDA) as a tissue bank.
c. Establish themselves as a nonprofit facility.
d. Store the tissue in pathology.

22. The critical danger sign(s) for a liver, biliary tract, pancreas, or spleen post-op patient to report to the physician is/are

a. fever of 38.3 °C (101 °F).
b. chills.
c. increased abdominal swelling or pain.
d. redness, swelling, and purulent drainage from the incision.

23. The Perioperative Patient Focused Model is divided into how many parts?

a. Three.
b. Four.
c. Six.
d. Eight.

24. The perioperative nurse records all of the following options when monitoring a patient who receives local anesthesia EXCEPT

a. skin color and condition.
b. blood pressure; pulse rate and rhythm; respirations; and O_2 saturation.
c. exact site of each local injection and time elapsed for anesthesia.
d. mental status; anesthetic dose; and temperature

25. Which of the following interventions would be LEAST effective to alleviate a patient's preoperative fear and anxiety?

a. Listen attentively.
b. Explain every detail of the proposed surgical procedure.
c. Provide reassurance.
d. Encourage her to express her anxiety and fear.

26. When the scrub RN is helping place the surgical drapes, he should be aware that once the drapes have been placed, they should not be moved or readjusted. Which of the following best describes the rationale for this placement?

a. Shifting of a drape can potentially cause contamination.
b. It reduces the cost of needing additional drapes.
c. Repositioning a drape is an acceptable practice.
d. Shifting of a drape can cause skin irritation.

27. The circulating RN is pouring sterile normal saline on the back field. She does not use all of the fluid in the container. Is it ok to recap the bottle and use the rest of the solution later on the field?

a. Yes, as long as the cap was kept sterile.
b. Yes, unless the OR's policy prohibits it.
c. No, because the edges of the container are not sterile.
d. It depends on the particular solution in the container.

28. While performing a Nissen fundoplication, the surgeon asks the nurse to place the bed in the reverse Trendelenburg position. Which of the following best describes this position?

a. Dorsal recumbent.
b. Supine with the head of the bed lower than the feet.
c. Supine with the head of the bed higher than the feet.
d. Supine with the patient's legs elevated in stirrups.

29. A nurse will be circulating a total knee replacement. He asks the surgeon to mark the site. Which of the following should be used to mark the surgical site?

a. A permanent skin marker.
b. A pen.
c. Any marker is appropriate, as long as the site is marked.
d. It is not necessary to mark the site, as long as the nurse has radiographs available.

30. There have been a lot of reports in the media regarding intraoperative awareness. Which of the following pieces of equipment can help the anesthesia care provider prevent this complication?

a. Electroencephalogram (EEG).
b. Electrocardiogram (EKG).
c. Bispectral index (BIS) monitoring.
d. Pulse oximetry.

31. If the external waist tie does not have a tag attached to it, what can it be placed in to pass it to the circulator?

a. Wrapped around a knife handle.
b. The paper packaging of the sterile gloves.
c. The ungloved hand of the surgeon.
d. The cuff of the gown.

32. The surgeon has ordered morphine sulfate (MS) for postoperative pain control. Which of the following is the most appropriate pediatric dosage?

a. 0.1-0.2 mg/kg IV.
b. 0.1-0.2 mg/kg PO.
c. 1-2 mg/kg IV.
d. 0.5-1 mg/kg IM.

33. A scrub nurse is preparing to scrub for a surgery. Which of the following is the best place for him to open his sterile gown and gloves so he can don them after his surgical scrub?

a. On the sterile back table.
b. On a separate sterile surface other than the back table.
c. On the sterile field.
d. Outside the OR suite.

34. A breast biopsy patient is tearful during the perioperative nursing assessment, so her most likely nursing diagnosis is

a. fear of body image change, pain, or death.
b. fear of medical personnel.
c. fear of anaphylactic reaction.
d. fear of missing work.

35. The most important piece of protective equipment used by OR personnel during a bronchoscopy is a

a. gown.
b. mask with shield and goggles.
c. gloves.
d. shoe covers.

36. During a perioperative assessment, the OR nurse notices a red rash under the Ace bandage on the patient's wrist, and around his IV insertion site, which delivers normal saline solution. The patient complains the area is itchy and the nurse hears him wheezing. The most likely problem is

a. possible latex allergy.
b. bronchitis.
c. hypersensitivity to IV solution.
d. psychological fear of surgery.

37. The length of surgical prep time is determined by

a. the OR Committee.
b. researchers who studied the effectiveness of the antimicrobial agents.
c. the manufacturer's recommendations.
d. the type of surgery being performed.

38. ER staff notifies the perioperative nurse at 03:00 to prepare for three critical MVA patients; two of them require simultaneous multiple procedures. The factors predisposing the surgical team to make wrong-site or wrong-patient errors include

a. emergency status, unusual time pressures, multiple surgeons, and simultaneous multiple procedures during a single session.
b. emergency status, multiple vehicle accidents, and time pressure to prepare the operating theaters.
c. unusual time pressures, multiple surgeons, and under-staffing.
d. unusual time for surgery, multiple theaters, and pressure for on-call staff.

39. A perioperative nurse observes a newly hired perioperative nurse remove his mask and pocket it for use in the next procedure, to save money. The best response to his action is

a. "Thanks for cost-saving. Just allow your mask to hang around your neck between procedures. Please don't put it in your pocket."
b. "Bag your used mask before you put it in your pocket. If you reuse your mask for cost-saving, don't contaminate it."
c. "Your mask is contaminated by microorganisms from your respiratory tract and from the procedure. Discard your mask after each procedure. Thanks for your concern, but safety surpasses saving money."
d. "Masks are expensive and your concern over cost-saving is admirable."

40. In which of the following procedures would a Javid shunt be utilized?

a. Thyroidectomy.
b. Aortic bifemoral bypass.
c. Carotid endarterectomy.
d. Cholecystectomy.

41. A nurse is circulating a trauma and requests packed red blood cells (PRBCs) to give to the patient in the OR suite. Unless the circulating nurse keeps the blood units in a cooler, how long can the units be out of the refrigerator before they cannot be returned to blood bank?

a. 10 minutes.
b. 30 minutes.
c. 1 hour.
d. 15 minutes.

42. A perioperative nurse dons a sterile gown and gloves, using the open glove technique. His scrubbed thumb touches the outside of his second sterile glove. The most appropriate next step is

a. continue gloving; his hand is bacteria-free, so he is uncontaminated.
b. discard the contaminated gloves and ask for new ones.
c. remove both his gown and gloves, then return to the scrub sink to start over.
d. continue gloving, and then rinse his hands in sterile saline.

43. When transfusing a patient in the PACU, the nurse suspects an adverse blood reaction. What is the first thing the PACU nurse should do?

a. Rush the blood in to prevent hypovolemia from the impending shock.
b. Send the unused blood to the blood bank.
c. Stop the transfusion.
d. Administer a bolus of normal saline.

44. A circulating RN is caring for a patient who is having a vaginal hysterectomy. After assisting the anesthesia care provider, the RN needs to place the patient's legs in stirrups. The nurse should always check with the anesthesia care provider to be sure it is safe to position the patient. Which of the following provides the best answer of why the patient should not be moved until the anesthesia provider says it is safe?

a. To give the anesthesia provider time to connect the vital sign monitors.
b. Because the patient may fall off the OR table if positioned without the other providers' awareness.
c. To prevent accidental extubation.
d. Because the anesthesia provider may still need to place invasive lines.

45. Which of the following is the minimum frequency that biological indicators should be run in the sterilizers?

a. Once a day.
b. Once a week and with all implants.
c. Once a month.
d. Bimonthly and with all implants.

46. What is bariatric surgery performed for?

a. Cancer.
b. Weight loss.
c. Fractures.
d. Renal failure.

47. The hospital administration has decided to implement shared governance but has found the nursing staff resistive because of the potential for the added work and extra time required during the development phase. The best recourse for the administration is to

a. impose a shared governance plan.
b. provide education and training about the process.
c. engage only key staff members in the process.
d. leave the details to an assigned committee.

48. An ever-present risk when giving general anesthesia is triggering a malignant hyperthermia (MH) incident. What is the test used to determine MH susceptibility?

a. Myoglobin urine test.
b. Allergy testing.
c. Caffeine-halothane contracture test.
d. Ab1 testing.

49. Which of the following is used as part of an active warming method?

a. Cotton blanket
b. Reflective blanket
c. Thermal clothing
d. Resistive polymer blanket

50. The cause of the majority of surgical site infections (SSI) is

a. poor aseptic technique.
b. the patient's own flora.
c. respiratory contaminants from perioperative personnel.
d. improperly cleaned lights in the operating theater.

51. Traffic into the OR suite should be limited. No unneeded personnel should be in the suite, and the staff should try to limit trips in and out of the room. What is the purpose of this traffic control?

a. It is one of several methods to limit microbes in the OR.
b. It is a security measure that is only used in emergency situations.
c. It keeps distractions to the team to a minimum.
d. Limitation of additional personnel in the OR suite is a safety measure the hospital institutes so there is less chance of injuries.

52. The scrub nurse is helping drape a patient for an appendectomy. She first drapes the area planned for the incision, and then she works outward. Why are surgical drapes laid in this manner?

a. To visually maintain the correct anatomical positioning of the patient.
b. To provide additional warmth during the surgical procedure.
c. To reduce contamination.
d. To verify that the correct site is being draped.

53. When circulating a laparoscopic surgery, the nurse sees the surgeon lay the light cord on the sterile drape. Which of the following would be the most effective action to prevent injury?

a. Turn off the endoscopic tower.
b. Turn the light on standby.
c. Tell the surgeon to move the light off the sterile drape.
d. Nothing needs to be done in this situation.

54. Which of the following is a therapeutic effect specific to midazolam hydrochloride (Versed)?

a. Nausea and vomiting.
b. Respiratory depression.
c. Short-term and retrograde amnesia.
d. Pain control.

55. A patient is scheduled for an arteriovenous (AV) fistula creation. She is a 62-year-old female with Type 1 diabetes. Which potential complication should the circulating nurse be aware of intraoperatively?

a. Infection.
b. Delayed wound healing.
c. Hypotension.
d. Hypertension.

56. A circulating RN is caring for an obese patient that needs to be placed in a right lateral position. Multiple staff members and the surgeon come in to help with proper positioning. Which of the following is the most important regarding documentation of positioning?

a. The number of people required to properly position.
b. Names of all team members and physicians involved with positioning the patient.
c. Preoperative skin condition.
d. Any invasive lines or drains that the patient came into the OR with.

57. Operating room bed mattresses are made of different materials. In reference to prevention of pressure injuries, which of the following is an effective OR table mattress material?

a. Foam.
b. Synthetic down.
c. Springs.
d. Gel.

58. Which of the following suture gauges is the smallest?

a. #0.
b. #5-0.
c. #11-0.
d. #2.

59. Whenever blood products are given to a patient, the correct information must be verified. Who can check blood products in the OR?

a. Anyone.
b. Only the surgeon and anesthesia care provider.
c. Any two licensed professionals.
d. Only the blood bank staff.

60. Which of the following sutures should not be used in an infected surgical site?

a. Gut.
b. Prolene.
c. Nylon.
d. Vicryl.

61. How should a pregnant patient in the supine position be positioned differently than a nonpregnant patient?

a. She should have a wedge placed under her left side.
b. She should have a pillow placed under her lower back.
c. She should have a wedge placed under her right side.
d. She should have a shoulder roll placed under her neck.

62. An example of a *never event* is

a. an appendix ruptures during surgery.
b. a surgery performed on the wrong body part.
c. simultaneous surgeries on multiple accident victims.
d. hemorrhage after surgery for a cerebral aneurysm.

63. What is the minimum number of staff members needed to safely transfer a patient who can assist?

a. 1.
b. 2.
c. 3.
d. 4.

64. Which of the following is an example of manual hemostasis?

a. Laser.
b. Fibrin glue.
c. Sutures.
d. Electrosurgical unit (ESU).

65. Now that the scrub nurse has properly grasped the sterile towel, which of the following best describes in which direction should she dry her hands and arms?

a. From the fingers upward toward the elbow, without going backward.
b. From the upper arm down to the fingers.
c. From the fingers upward toward the elbow and then back down.
d. Upward from one hand to the other, and then both forearms.

66. A circulating nurse's patient was in a motor vehicle accident, and, unfortunately, he does not survive. Which outside department should the circulating nurse call to report the patient's death?

a. Fire department.
b. Media.
c. Coroner's office.
d. Funeral home.

67. What is the difference between chemical and biological indicators?

a. Chemical indicators indicate sterility for instruments, and biological indicators are for implants.
b. Both indicate sterility but for different agents, chemical for chemical and biological for radiation.
c. Chemical indicators do not ensure sterility and only show that the parameters of the sterilizer have been met, but biological indicators test for actual sterility through the use of resistant spores.
d. Chemical indicators ensure sterility of instruments, and biological indicators test for proper function of the autoclaves.

68. In which of the following surgeries would the scrub nurse possibly use 3% sorbitol as a fluid media?

a. Hysteroscopy.
b. Laparoscopic cholecystectomy.
c. Cystoscopy.
d. Laparoscopic salpingo-oophorectomy.

69. Unsterile personnel, such as the circulating RN, should stay away from the sterile field to avoid contamination. Which of the following is the minimum distance an unsterile person should remain from the sterile field?

a. 15 in.
b. 6 in.
c. 12 cm.
d. 1 ft.

70. A patient become hypotensive during surgery. The surgeon verbally orders the nurse to administer a 500 mL bolus of Lactated Ringer solution. The correct verification method is to

a. write the order on a paper or white board; show it to the surgeon for confirmation.
b. confirm it with the scrub nurse.
c. check the patient's record for drug allergies.
d. check the patient's record for drug orders.

71. In addition to surgical site marking, a "time out" is performed by the surgical team to ensure the right patient and planned procedure is agreed upon. When should this process take place?

a. In the preoperative holding area.
b. Immediately before the procedure.
c. After the surgeon makes the incision.
d. Prior to draping the patient.

72. A scrub nurse has finished scrubbing a surgery and is breaking down his sterile field. What does he do with his surgical sharps, such as suture needles?

a. Place them in a biohazard bag.
b. Place them in a puncture-proof sharps container.
c. Place them in a puncture-proof box to be resterilized.
d. Place them in a regular trash bag.

73. When conducting a surgery using a laser, how should the laser be handled when not in use?

a. Turn it off.
b. Place it on standby.
c. Be sure it is not facing any team members.
d. No special handling is required.

74. When placing sterile drapes around the surgical site to create the sterile field, how should the drapes be held?

a. Higher than the OR table and placed from the surgical site outward.
b. Higher than the OR table and placed from the outside in toward the surgical site.
c. Under the OR table and brought around the patient.
d. It does not matter as long as the scrub nurse does not touch anything nonsterile with the sterile drapes.

75. If a nonsterile equipment item is to be used in the sterile field, such as a C-arm device or ultrasound Doppler, what is the best way to use it and protect the surgical wound?

a. The equipment should be covered with a sterile drape.
b. It does not need to be draped because the field is already sterile.
c. No special handling is required because is not a contamination risk.
d. Simply cover the surgical site with a sterile towel when using the nonsterile equipment.

76. The Joint Commission's targeted solution for reducing patient injuries that result from poor communication between caregivers is

a. a standardized hand-off procedure.
b. preoperative instructions for patients to read.
c. safety standards for Holding Area staff.
d. marking the surgical site.

77. When preparing to perform a skin prep on a patient who is having an autologous skin graft placed over a debrided ulcer site on her right foot, the surgeon has informed the scrub nurse that the donor site will be the patient's left thigh. Which of the following best describes how the nurse should perform the surgical skin prep for this patient?

a. He should use one prep set, prepping the recipient site and then the donor site.
b. He needs to prep the recipient site but not the donor site, because he is only removing skin from that area.
c. He should first prep the donor site using a colorless prep, and then prep the recipient site.
d. He should first prep the recipient site using a colorless prep, and then prep the donor site.

78. It is imperative for the surgical team to keep track of sponges and instruments used during the surgery so that items are not inadvertently left in a patient. Which three positions and in which order should closing counts be performed?

a. Field, floor (off the sterile field), back table.
b. Back table, floor, field.
c. Initial, baseline, final.
d. Field, back table, floor.

79. The American Society of Anesthesiologists (ASA) status III would apply to which of the following patients?

a. Healthy patient.
b. Mild systemic disease.
c. Brain death.
d. Severe systemic disease.

80. Which of the following is a discharge assessment area in Phase I of PACU but not in Phase II?

a. Airway patency.
b. Nausea level.
c. Level of consciousness.
d. Motor and sensory function.

81. The areas of expertise essential for the perioperative nurse include all of the following EXCEPT

a. anatomy.
b. endotracheal tube insertion and internal physical landmarks.
c. perioperative safety.
d. surgical procedures, instruments, and equipment.

82. The responsibility of the circulating nurse to the patient's family when surgery is prolonged is

a. the only obligations are to the patient.
b. call into the Waiting Room to inform the family about the patient's condition, and to relay updates from the surgeon.
c. go to the Waiting Room in person to check on the family and to give them updates.
d. go to the waiting room to offer the family coffee.

83. The perioperative nurse is helping place a patient in the lateral position for a right thoracotomy surgery. The nurse should be aware of the potential for which injury with this type of position?

a. Lower back strain.
b. Pressure injuries to the posterior skull.
c. Nerve damage to the extremities.
d. Skin tears on the buttocks.

84. An older patient who is quite weak after a recent total knee replacement surgery will have nursing care and physical therapy through a home health agency. The patient has limited income and believes that she can manage independently but is concerned about cooking. What is the best recommendation to give her?

a. Sit on a stool while cooking.
b. Use frozen meals that can be microwaved.
c. Ask friends or family to assist with meals.
d. Encourage her to apply for Meals on Wheels.

85. Which of the following is a true statement regarding sponge counts?

a. Sponge counts only need to be done before and after the procedure.
b. Sponge counts should be done whenever any team member leaves the room.
c. As long as the sponge count is performed at wound closure, the scrub nurse does not need to count for each cavity closure.
d. Sponge counts should be done at any permanent relief of either the scrub or circulating nurse.

86. What is a dermatome device used for?

a. Removing valves from a vein graft.
b. Promoting bone growth in nonhealing fractures.
c. Removing tissue to be used in split-thickness skin grafts.
d. Locating sentinel lymph nodes.

87. ViaSpan is used in which of the following procedures?

a. Coronary artery bypass graft (CABG) surgery.
b. Heart catheterization.
c. Living-donor nephrectomy.
d. Pancreas transplant.

88. The preoperative nurse knows her patient, who is a smoker, has additional healthcare risks to take in account when planning his plan of care. Compared to the other patients, what are smokers' risks for developing pressure injuries during a long surgical procedure?

a. They are at higher risk for pressure injury formation.
b. They are at lower risk for pressure injury formation.
c. They are at the same risk for pressure injury formation.
d. They are not at any risk for pressure injuries because smoking causes vasodilatation.

89. What is the recommended dose range for IV dantrolene?

a. 1.5 mg/kg initially, up to 15 mg/kg.
b. 0.25 mg/kg initially, up to 10 mg/kg.
c. 1.5 mg/lb initially, up to 50 mg/lb.
d. 2.5 mg/kg initially, up to 10 mg/kg.

90. The drug of choice for malignant hyperthermia patients is

a. dantrolene sodium (Dantrium).
b. succinylcholine (Anectine).
c. fentanyl.
d. morphine.

91. Why is spinal cord damage an operative risk with thoracic aortic aneurysm repair?

a. Because the spinal cord may be cut in the procedure.
b. Because the spinal cord may experience ischemia if the cross-clamp time is excessive.
c. Because these patients are at high risk of stroke.
d. Because these patients often have already had spine surgery.

92. The Kraske position would be appropriate for which of the following procedures?

a. Total vaginal hysterectomy.
b. Total abdominal hysterectomy.
c. Rectal surgery.
d. Thyroidectomy.

93. Which of the following is one of the most commonly used medications for epidural anesthesia?

a. Meperidine.
b. Bacitracin.
c. Bupivacaine.
d. Succinylcholine.

94. Surgical team members who are routinely exposed to procedures using x rays, such as orthopedic cases, and are less than two feet away from the radiation beam should wear which of the following additional protective items?

a. Thyroid shield.
b. Eye protection.
c. Laser mask.
d. Wrap-around lead aprons.

95. The circulating RN on a laparoscopic cholecystectomy sees the suction tip is extending off the edge of the sterile back table but has not fallen off. What should the circulating nurse do?

a. Tell the scrub tech so she can move it back on the table before it falls.
b. Tell the scrub tech to discard the tip.
c. Nothing: as long as it's still on the table, it's still sterile.
d. Remove it from the back table herself.

96. Following a large Formalin spill on her surgical scrubs, the resource a perioperative nurse must look to in order to find out its hazards and appropriate first aid is

a. OSHA.
b. SDS.
c. NIOSH.
d. FDA.

97. The anesthesia care provider has informed the scrub nurse she will be performing a Bier block on the patient. Which piece of equipment would be necessary to perform this procedure?

a. Electrosurgical unit (ESU).
b. Single-cuff tourniquet.
c. Double-cuff tourniquet.
d. BIS monitor.

98. In order to prevent injury to fellow team members, the scrub RN should pass loaded knife blades in which of the following manners?

a. With the blade toward the physician.
b. With the blade off the handle.
c. With a "hands-free" technique.
d. With the blade in his/her hand.

99. In elderly patients, why would the perioperative nurses want to carefully monitor which medications the patient is given postoperatively?

a. Drug tolerance can be very high in the elderly due to the large number of medications they may regularly take.
b. Elderly patients metabolize anesthesia medications very quickly and will require larger doses of pain medications for comfort.
c. Elderly patients have many more drug allergies.
d. Elderly patients are more prone to drug interactions because they have lower tolerance and excretion of medications.

100. When circulating a carotid endarterectomy, and the surgeon asks for loupes. What is she asking for?

a. Vessel loops.
b. Her magnifying eyeglasses.
c. Silk ties.
d. Hemaclips.

101. The general recommendation for hair at the surgical site is to:

a. leave it in place
b. shave it
c. remove it with clippers
d. remove it with a depilatory

102. Once the patient is brought into the surgical suite and transferred from her gurney to the OR table, what should the scrub nurse do?

a. A safety strap is placed over her thighs.
b. A staff member stays and holds her in place.
c. No safety strap is necessary because the patient is not sedated.
d. A safety strap is placed across the chest.

103. Class 2 therapeutic compression stockings are commonly used as VTE prophylaxis. They provide pressure of:

a. 40–50 mmHg
b. 30–40 mmHg
c. 20–30 mmHg
d. 10–20 mmHg

104. There are three types of blood loss replacements used in the perioperative setting. Autotransfusion is an example of which one of the following?

a. Allogenous blood transfusion.
b. Autologous blood transfusion.
c. Blood product substitution.
d. Blood volume expander.

105. A circulating RN's patient is having an exploratory laparotomy in the supine position. When the patient is in a supine position with arms extended, how should his palms be placed?

a. They should face up (supination).
b. They should face down (pronation).
c. Positioning the hands is not important.
d. They should be placed lateral facing toward the body.

106. What Aldrete score would the nurse give a recovering postoperative total hip replacement patient if she is fully awake and moving all extremities, her blood pressure is being maintained at her preoperative state, but she is having difficulty breathing deeply, and her O_2 saturation is 92% with 2L oxygen per nasal cannula?

a. 10.
b. 6.
c. 8.
d. 9.

107. Even though a Mexican immigrant patient obviously appears to be in pain (i.e., grimacing, moaning, in the fetal position) after major surgery, when asked to quantify the pain on a 1–10 scale, the patient repeatedly says "1." What is the most appropriate intervention?

a. Ask the patient to describe the pain in a different way.
b. Withhold medication because the patient's pain is mild.
c. Withhold medication and assume that the patient is avoiding pain medication.
d. Administer pain medication because the patient appears to be in pain.

108. Which of the following is an example of an antiseptic solution often found as an ingredient in surgical skin preps?

a. Chlorhexidine gluconate.
b. Acetone.
c. Water.
d. ChloraPrep.

109. The circulating RN should verify that the anesthesia provider has given preoperative antibiotics as ordered by the surgeon. In what time frame should these be given for a patient who is not already on routine antibiotics?

a. 24 hours before the surgical incision.
b. 6 hours before the surgical incision.
c. 1 hour before the surgical incision.
d. 2 days after the surgery.

110. Which of the following would be an appropriate environmental safety precaution when performing procedures utilizing lasers?

a. Placing warning signs outside the OR suite that a laser is being used.
b. Removing all fluids from the surgical area so they do not spill on the laser.
c. Keeping the laser armed at all times so it is ready when needed.
d. Keeping an ABC-type fire extinguisher in the room.

111. What does a reading of 100 on the BIS monitor means?

a. The patient is fully awake.
b. The patient is highly sedated.
c. The patient is clinically brain dead.
d. The BIS monitoring machine is malfunctioning.

112. To prevent hypothermia, IV fluids are typically warmed to a maximum temperature of:

a. 95 °F (35 °C)
b. 98.7 °F (37 °C)
c. 106 °F (41 °C)
d. 111 °F (44 °C)

113. What does the acronym ESWL stand for?

a. External shock wave ligation.
b. Extracorporeal shock wave ligation.
c. Extracorporeal shock wave lithotripsy.
d. External shock wave lithotripsy.

114. In which of the following procedures might a Litvak Pereyra needle be used?

a. Spinal anesthesia.
b. Abdominal aortic aneurysm repair.
c. Bladder neck suspension.
d. Epidural anesthesia.

115. The nursing process is essential in developing a perioperative plan of care. This six-part process includes assessment, nursing diagnosis, identifying outcomes, implementation, evaluation, and

a. benchmarking.
b. planning.
c. communicating.
d. interventions.

116. Surgical specimens are listed according to three categories for handling. Which of the following best describes these categories?

a. Surgical pathology, gross, disposal.
b. Frozen, permanent, gross.
c. Frozen, permanent, disposal.
d. Banking, surgical pathology, disposal.

117. The circulating RN must assist the surgeon with placement of his sterile gown. Which of the following is true regarding what area the circulator may touch on the surgeon's gown?

a. The external waist tie.
b. The wrist ties.
c. The internal waist ties.
d. None of the ties.

118. What is the difference between the semirestricted and restricted areas of the operating room department?

a. In the semirestricted areas, surgical personnel can wear street clothes, but in the restricted area, they must wear surgical scrubs.
b. Both areas require surgical personnel to wear surgical scrubs, but in the restricted area they must wear a hair covering.
c. There is no semirestricted area in the operating room, just an unrestricted and restricted.
d. In both areas, surgical personnel must wear scrubs and a hair cover, but in the restricted areas, they must also wear a surgical mask.

119. The circulating RN knows that using proper draping materials is essential for patient protection. Which of the following best describes the current recommendations for choosing the correct draping material?

a. The drapes must be resistant to fluid, tearing, puncture, and lint free to reduce contamination of the sterile field.
b. Different institutions decide on the guidelines that best suit their organizational needs and policies.
c. The current recommendations are under review, and they will be available in the upcoming year.
d. The drapes must be able to maintain the heat of the human body to avoid hypothermia during the surgical procedure.

120. The scrub nurse pulls up which part of the gown when assisting the surgeon in gloving?

a. The shoulder of the gown.
b. The waist of the gown.
c. The sleeves of the gown.
d. The neck of the gown.

121. Which of the following spores is the most resistant?

a. Viral.
b. Bacterial.
c. Fungal.
d. Tuberculosis.

122. The Kraske position is also known as which of the following?

a. Lithotomy.
b. Supine.
c. Jackknife.
d. Lateral.

123. Which of the following is a type of chemical sterilizing agent?

a. Steam.
b. Ethylene oxide.
c. Microwave.
d. X ray.

124. To ensure the patient remains free of infection, the OR nurse must use all of the following methods EXCEPT

a. excellent aseptic technique.
b. proper preparation for the incision site.
c. proper draping methods.
d. proper anesthesia.

125. The main modes of transmission for microorganisms in the OR are

a. droplet, airborne, and contact.
b. body fluids, purulent material, and blood.
c. sneezing, coughing, and talking.
d. blood and dirty equipment.

126. A nurse is performing her preoperative assessment on a 68-year-old male who is scheduled for an elective coronary artery bypass graft (CABG) surgery. Which of the following home medications should the patient not have stopped before surgery?

a. Plavix.
b. Warfarin.
c. Lasix.
d. Aspirin.

127. Following a surgical procedure, a patient develops premature ventricular contractions (PVCs). Which electrolyte imbalance may be implicated?

a. Hypercalcemia.
b. Hypocalcemia.
c. Hypokalemia.
d. Hyperkalemia.

128. If a pneumatic tourniquet is used for more than 75 minutes on a pediatric patient, the patient should be assessed for:

a. acidosis
b. petechiae
c. alkalosis
d. nerve injury

129. When the surgeon is marking a surgical site, which of the following methods is most appropriate?

a. Placing an X on the surgical site.
b. Writing YES on the surgical site.
c. Writing NO on the nonsurgical site.
d. Placing an X on the nonsurgical site.

130. Laparoscopic surgeries, such as laparoscopic cholecystectomy, require gas to be infused in the abdomen. The following three questions refer to this type of surgery. What type of gas is used?

a. Argon.
b. Carbon dioxide.
c. Carbon monoxide.
d. Nitrogen.

131. The coroner has released a deceased patient, and the circulating nurse is preparing to transfer him to the morgue. Where should the circulating nurse place the patient's identification tags before transport?

a. On the patient and on the chart, anywhere visible.
b. On the patient and the shroud.
c. Only one tag is needed on the gurney transporting the patient.
d. As long as the patient has an identification armband, he does not need additional identification tags.

132. Which of the following items should not be used in the surgical wound?

a. Lap sponges.
b. Ray-Tec sponges.
c. Radiopaque towels.
d. Nonradiopaque towels.

133. A nurse has removed a warm bottle of normal saline from his facility's fluid warmer. At the end of the surgery, he did not use the fluid. What should he do with it?

a. Put it back in the warmer.
b. Change the expiration date to account for the time it was removed from the warmer.
c. Label the bottle "Do Not Rewarm," and store at room temperature.
d. Discard it.

134. Which of the following patients would be a candidate for bariatric surgery?

a. A 40-year-old female with a BMI of 30 with mild comorbidities.
b. A 45-year-old male with a BMI of 45 and no other complications.
c. A 30-year-old female with a BMI of 35 with no other complications.
d. None of the above patients are candidates for this surgery.

135. For which piece of the following equipment should the scrub nurse place a return electrode on the patient?

a. Electrosurgical unit (ESU).
b. Greenlight laser.
c. Ultrasonic dissector.
d. Flexible endoscope.

136. Which of the following bariatric surgeries is a combination of the restrictive and malabsorption methods?

a. Gastric banding.
b. Proximal gastric bypass.
c. Roux-en-Y gastric bypass.
d. Jejunoileal bypass.

137. A postanesthesia care RN is recovering a new postoperative open appendectomy patient. How frequently should the RN monitor vital signs in the initial postoperative period in the PACU?

a. Every 5 minutes.
b. Every 15 minutes.
c. Every 30 minutes.
d. Every 60 minutes.

138. The magnetic field of an MRI scan is considered safe for the general public beyond the:

a. 2 gauss line
b. 4 gauss line
c. 5 gauss line
d. 7 gauss line

139. A nurse is circulating a surgery, and the planned position is prone. Which of the following would be appropriate equipment needed for this type of positioning?

a. Chest rolls/bolsters.
b. Stirrups.
c. Footboard.
d. Vacuum-assisted positioning device (beanbag).

140. In order to lower the risk of surgical site infections, the doors to the OR suite should remain in which of the following positions?

a. Open if a surgery is in process.
b. Closed as much as possible.
c. Open if there is no surgery occurring.
d. The position of the OR doors does not affect infection control.

141. The circulating nurse is in an orthopedic procedure utilizing a C-arm device when the surgeon asks for this device to be moved to another area of the patient's body. Which of the following personnel may move this device?

a. Only the circulating RN.
b. Any MD.
c. The orthopedic vendor.
d. The radiology tech.

142. In which areas is the scrub nurse considered sterile after donning a sterile gown and gloves?

a. Everywhere covered by the gown.
b. Only the hands.
c. From the chest to the sterile field.
d. Front and back of gown, chest to waist.

143. The primary purpose of the read-back procedure when taking a verbal or telephone order is to

a. ensure the accuracy of the order.
b. comply with regulations.
c. save time.
d. show that you are paying attention.

144. In order to ensure proper functioning of the anesthesia monitoring equipment, patients should be informed to remove which of the following before surgery?

a. Jewelry.
b. Glasses.
c. Dentures.
d. Nail polish and acrylic nails.

145. The disadvantage(s) of using rigid containers to hold sterile instruments include all of the following EXCEPT

a. weight.
b. instrument damage.
c. residual condensation.
d. contamination.

146. In relation to surgical attire, which of the following is correct?

a. It should be flammable.
b. It should always be disposable.
c. It should be low linting.
d. It can be reworn if not soiled.

147. When circulating a laparoscopic cholecystectomy, and the surgeon asks the circulating nurse for a Veress needle. What is the purpose of this device?

a. To insert local anesthetic into the surgical field.
b. To insufflate the abdominal cavity.
c. To aspirate the gallbladder.
d. To insert the trocar into the abdominal cavity.

148. Which of the following is a monofilament absorbable suture?

a. Chromic gut.
b. Polypropylene.
c. Nylon.
d. Vicryl.

149. The circulating nurse does NOT document

a. amount of prep solution.
b. type and amount of irrigation.
c. fluid output.
d. blood products.

150. An 18-year-old patient who has been deaf since birth has recently received cochlear implants. When communicating with this patient, it is essential to

a. face the patient and speak slowly.
b. use gestures and notes to supplement speech.
c. ask if the patient needs a sign language interpreter.
d. speak normally.

151. A 1-day-old neonate is to undergo emergency surgery but has an elevated total bilirubin level. What total bilirubin level is considered critical in the newborn?

a. >13 mg/dL.
b. >10 mg/dL.
c. >7 mg/dL.
d. >5 mg/dL.

152. The information regarding the patient's position that the nurse must document is

a. skin condition before and after surgery; type and placement of positioning equipment; team members who positioned the patient; and changes in position.
b. height of the operating table and Mayo stand.
c. number of perioperative staff assisting the surgeon.
d. A and B.

153. A PACU nurse is recovering a patient after an aortic valve replacement surgery. Which of the following is the most common cardiac arrhythmia after this type of surgery?

a. Bradycardia.
b. Tachycardia.
c. Atrial fibrillation.
d. Heart block.

154. When changing a surgical dressing, the nurse notes a small, firm, slightly erythematous raised area along one part of the incision; this is most likely a(n)

a. rash.
b. dehiscence.
c. ecchymosis.
d. hematoma.

155. The room temperature in the operating room suites must be maintained within a specific range. Which one of the following answers provides the correct temperature range?

a. 68-73 °F.
b. 65-70 °F.
c. 55-60 °F.
d. 65-75 °F.

156. Mrs. Smith is scheduled for an endovascular procedure. She is allergic to shellfish. Which of the following could be affected by this allergy?

a. Antibiotic choice.
b. Use of latex products.
c. Use of contrast media.
d. Administration of Propofol.

157. A patient develops hypothermia (with a temperature of 35 °C [95 °F]). Despite active warming with forced-air blankets, the patient begins to experience severe shivering. Which one of the following drugs is most often used to reduce shivering?

a. Meperidine.
b. Doxapram.
c. Alfentanil.
d. Morphine.

158. One of the factors in determining a patient's acuity score is the length of the surgery time. After how much time in the same position is the patient's injury risk increased?

a. 1 hour.
b. 2 hours.
c. 3 hours.
d. 0.5 hours.

159. A patient is scheduled for a decortication of the right lung. What does this mean?

a. A lobe of the right lung is going to be removed.
b. Restrictive tissue is going to be stripped from this lung.
c. A chest tube is going to be placed to remove fluid from the right lung.
d. A wedge biopsy is going to be performed on this lung.

160. The steam sterilizer has finished its cycle. What should a nurse working in the sterile processing department (SPD) do with these sterile items?

a. Unload them and leave them to dry on a table for 30 minutes.
b. Open the door of the sterilizer, and leave the products inside to dry for 15 to 60 minutes.
c. Unload the items and up them away immediately, so there is no inadvertent contamination.
d. Place the sterilizer on the drying cycle.

161. The purpose of aseptic practice is to do all of the following EXCEPT

a. to sterilize the skin by eliminating all bacteria.
b. to prevent contamination of an open wound with infectious agents.
c. to maintain a sterile field isolated from the adjacent unsterilized area.
d. to minimize the risk of infection during surgery.

162. Which of the following is an intravenous general anesthetic commonly given to children?

a. Versed.
b. Demerol.
c. Ketamine.
d. Suprane.

163. Suture needles are categorized as three types: cutting, blunt, and tapered. How many variations of these types are there?

a. 3.
b. 5.
c. 6.
d. 10.

164. Which of the following single-use items should not be reprocessed?

a. Sutures.
b. Trocars.
c. Endoscopic graspers.
d. Opened and unused staplers.

165. Which of the following medications is LEAST relevant in the operating room?

a. Dantrolene.
b. Propofol.
c. Succinylcholine.
d. Lasix.

166. With a unidirectional ultraclean air delivery system in use, which of the following should be within the air curtain?

a. The surgical site
b. The surgical site and instrument tables
c. The surgical site, lights, and microscopes
d. The surgical site and microscopes

167. Many medications are administered during the perioperative phase. The five "rights" of safe medication administration include right patient, drug, dose, route, and which of the following?

a. Method.
b. Physician.
c. Time.
d. Order.

168. A circulating RN should be aware of possible complications that may occur during the procedure. Which of the following is the most common potential complication of femoropopliteal (fem-pop) bypass surgery?

a. Renal damage from the on-table angiograms.
b. Nerve damage.
c. Operative leg swelling.
d. Femoral artery aneurysm.

169. The exogenous sources of infection include all of the following EXCEPT

a. cracks in nail polish, artificial nails, and jewelry.
b. talking, coughing, and breathing.
c. the patient's skin flora.
d. contaminated surgical instruments or supplies.

170. Which of the following describes a special consideration for correct draping that the scrub and circulating RN should be aware of?

a. They should ensure that the prep solutions have dried before applying surgical drapes.
b. The scrubbed team members should hold the drapes below waist level.
c. The surgeon should perform the procedure quickly to minimize potential infections.
d. The scrubbed team members never cuff the drapes over gloved hands.

171. Which of the following is the most important reason to record the amount of fluid infused and the amount returned during a hysteroscopy?

a. So the patient does not get an infection.
b. To prevent a distended bladder.
c. Because fluids can be absorbed and cause severe complications.
d. To correctly determine blood loss.

172. What is the purpose of introducing gas into the abdomen during laparoscopic surgeries?

a. Better visualization of internal structures.
b. Control bleeding.
c. Compress internal organs.
d. To give the surgeon a method to insert instruments into abdomen.

173. A nurse is recovering a patient in the PACU who had a malignant hyperthermia event in the operating room. How long after the original MH episode must the patient receive dantrolene intravenously?

a. 1-2 hours.
b. 24-72 hours.
c. 8-12 hours.
d. 5 days.

174. Which of the following best describes the difference between turnover OR suite cleaning and terminal OR suite cleaning?

a. Turnover is done at the beginning and terminal at the end of the day.
b. Terminal is cleaning between each case, and turnover is done at the end of the day.
c. Terminal cleaning is the thorough cleaning done at the end of the day, while turnover is the cleaning done between cases.
d. These two terms mean the same thing and are interchangeable.

175. Beck's triad is made up of high jugular venous pressure, low arterial pressure, and quiet heart sounds. These symptoms are indicative of which syndrome?

a. Increased intracranial pressure.
b. Pneumothorax.
c. Acute cardiac tamponade.
d. Cardiac asystole.

176. The standard criterion for sterile packaging material is that it must

a. resist tears, punctures, and abrasions.
b. prevent infiltration and egress of sterilant.
c. be waterproof.
d. be puncture-proof.

177. Which of the following is the recommended abdominal pressure during laparoscopic cases?

a. 30-45 mmHg.
b. 12-15 mmHg.
c. 5-10 mmHg.
d. 20-28 mmHg.

178. After the surgical scrub, if the scrub nurse is not using an alcohol-based scrub product, she will need to dry her hands. Which of the following is the best method to pick up the sterile towel?

a. Unfold it with both hands.
b. By the corner, with one hand.
c. In the middle, with one hand.
d. It does not matter how she picks up the towel.

179. Immediately before beginning any procedure, what should the circulating nurse do?

a. Call a "time out" with all team members involved with the procedure.
b. Identity the patient.
c. Find sitting stools.
d. Start an IV line.

180. Forensic specimens, such as bullets, should be carefully handled and properly documented to preserve which of the following?

a. Chain of evidence.
b. Chain of command.
c. Chain of communication.
d. Chain of custody.

181. In which magnetic resonance imaging (MRI) scan zone is the patient screened and prepared for an intraoperative MRI scan?

a. Zone I
b. Zone II
c. Zone III
d. Zone IV

182. The most commonly used preservative for biological specimens is:

a. 10% formalin
b. 20% formalin
c. 30% formalin
d. 40% formalin

183. What is the purpose of a UNOS number?

a. It is used for surgical billing.
b. It is used to identify appropriate bone implants assigned during a surgery.
c. It is the anonymous number given to trauma patients.
d. It is the identification number assigned to living and cadaver transplant organs.

184. Which of the following is the appropriate way to warm irrigation fluids?

a. Microwave.
b. Autoclave.
c. Warming cabinet or portable fluid warmer.
d. Warm blanket.

185. When transporting a three-year old female to the operating room for an appendectomy, the circulating nurse might expect her to demonstrate which behavior?

a. Concerns for physical appearance after the surgery.
b. Crying for parents.
c. Pretends to be Wonder Woman.
d. Nonverbal sounds only.

186. When should the scrub nurse perform an instrument count in addition to sponge and sharp counts?

a. Only on abdominal cases.
b. Only on trauma cases.
c. Any time there is a risk of a retained instrument.
d. Instrument counts are never necessary.

187. The critical value for the blood urea nitrogen level of an adult patient is

a. >35 mg/dL.
b. >55 mg/dL.
c. >100 mg/dL.
d. >120 mg/dL.

188. A Maryland dissector forceps would most commonly be used in which of the following surgeries?

a. Lumbar laminectomy.
b. Vaginal hysterectomy.
c. Laparoscopic cholecystectomy.
d. Thyroidectomy.

189. Which of the following complications is associated with thoracotomy but not video-assisted thoracoscopy (VAT)?

a. Infection.
b. Spinal cord injury.
c. Bleeding.
d. Pneumothorax.

190. The circulating RN is preparing for a hysteroscopy. The surgeon has requested Dextran as the fluid media. Which of the following would be a potential contraindication to using this fluid?

a. Monopolar electrosurgery.
b. Renal disease.
c. Allergy to shellfish.
d. Allergy to beet sugar.

191. What is the primary purpose of wearing surgical attire?

a. To distinguish to the patient who is the surgical RN.
b. To prevent bacterial shedding.
c. To act as personal protective equipment.
d. To prevent the spread of communicable diseases.

192. If using a gas-powered pneumatic tourniquet, which of the following is an appropriate gas to use?

a. Compressed air.
b. Carbon dioxide.
c. Nitrous oxide.
d. Oxygen.

193. When scrubbing an exploratory laparotomy, the scrub nurse places an instrument magnet pad on the sterile field to prevent the instruments from falling. Which of the following should the nurse not place on the instrument magnet?

a. Needle holder.
b. Tenaculum clamp.
c. Mayo scissor.
d. Poole suction tip.

194. The proper tape for a sterile pack is

a. surgical adhesive tape.
b. pressure-sensitive, striped chemical indicator tape.
c. double-sided paper tape.
d. extra-strength water resistant tape.

195. A circulating RN is caring for a patient receiving a carpal tunnel release under a brachial nerve block. When the circulating nurse documents the type of anesthesia, she should list which of the following?

a. General anesthesia.
b. Epidural anesthesia.
c. Regional anesthesia.
d. Monitored anesthesia care.

196. How does the phrase "event-related" apply to supplies in the operating room?

a. Package integrity.
b. Surgical time.
c. Surgical type.
d. Bulk sales from vendors.

197. What should the circulating RN do while the anesthesia care provider is intubating the patient during general anesthesia?

a. Stay by the head of the bed and assist as needed.
b. Leave the room to get supplies.
c. Help the scrub nurse count instruments.
d. Start her charting.

198. In regard to marking a surgical site when a side is specified, which of the following persons should mark the surgical site?

a. The patient.
b. The preoperative RN.
c. The circulating RN.
d. The surgeon.

199. The responsibilities of the perioperative nurse include all of the following EXCEPT

a. assessing the patient and developing the nursing diagnosis.
b. identifying desired outcomes and evaluating care.
c. developing and executing a discharge plan.
d. implementing the plan of care.

200. Which if the following is NOT a responsibility of the circulating nurse?

a. Transporting the patient into the Operating Room.
b. Taking report from the Holding Area nurse.
c. Relaying patient information to other perioperative staff.
d. Passing instruments to the surgeon during surgery.

Answer Key and Explanations for Test #2

1. C: Cricoid pressure helps block the esophagus to prevent aspiration of gastric contents. This would be especially important for a patient with a history of gastroesophageal reflux disease (GERD), because he would be at additional risk of aspiration. Cricoid has no purpose in keeping the neck stable. Closing off the esophagus actually helps the anesthesia care provider better visualize the vocal cords, a necessary landmark when intubating a patient with an endotracheal (ET) tube.

2. D: Hyperkalemia is a serious side effect of MH. It can cause serious cardiac dysrhythmias and renal damage. Using fluids containing potassium will increase the already-elevated serum potassium levels, causing further serious side effects.

3. A: Versed is a benzodiazepine. Romazicon, also known as Flumazenil, is the only benzodiazepine antagonist in this group. Narcan, also known as Naloxone hydrochloride, would be appropriate for narcotic reversal. Although Benadryl might be helpful for an allergic reaction, it will not reverse the effects of a benzodiazepine. Epinephrine would be helpful in an arrest situation as well, but it will not reverse the effects either.

4. B: If the nurse will be gowning and gloving herself, she should not open her supplies on the back table, in order to prevent contamination. It is acceptable to open these supplies on the back table if someone else, who is already wearing sterile supplies, will assist her so she is not required to touch the sterile back table to retrieve her supplies.

5. B: One of the risks of a carotid endarterectomy is possible damage to the nerves that control the movement of the vocal cords. Paralysis of the vocal cords can cause many complications, including difficulty breathing.

6. B: This is the recommended method by perioperative professional organizations to open sterile items. Loose edges could fold back and contaminate the instrument or field because the inside wrapper is only considered sterile up to 1 inch from the edge. As a result, the person opening should keep control of the flaps in her hand as she opens. In this question, the scrub tech is already sterile, so she cannot open the instrument because the outside of the wrap is not sterile.

7. A: A fenestrated drape is the formal name for a drape with openings. These openings can be in a variety of shapes and in multiple locations.

8. B: The patient return electrode "grounds" the patient from injury from the ESU current. Poor contact can prevent this function and even allow fluid to pool underneath it, leading to a possible burn. The tip of the ESU pencil can remain very hot between uses. Laying this tip on a surgical drape may start a fire. The ESU pencil should always be returned to its holder between uses. The patient return electrode should not be placed over a previous surgical site, if possible, because the electrical current could conduct through any metal implant that might exist at the site, or the tissue may already be compromised from poor wound healing. Finally, evidence-based practice shows alcohol-based preps to be very effective in the prevention of surgical site infections. It is safe to use this type of prep in the operating room as long as the manufacturer's recommendations are followed and the prep is dried completely before the surgical drape is applied.

9. A: Infection, hemorrhage, pneumothorax, and recurrent laryngeal nerve injury are all possible complications of mediastinoscopic surgery.

10. D: The nurse would want to slowly release the tourniquet so the body can absorb any remaining local anesthesia. A bolus of this medication could lead to cardiac or central nervous system toxicity. There should not be excessive bleeding or pain with this type of anesthesia.

11. D: Of the parts listed, the umbilicus is considered a contaminated area. If it will be included in the surgical field, such as an abdominal surgery, it should be prepped first; otherwise, contaminates could be dragged out and disrupt the already-prepped site. In this case, surgical swabs soaked in appropriate surgical prep are usually used to clean the umbilicus, and then the rest of the abdomen is prepped.

12. D: Laryngeal nerve paralysis is a possible complication when administering a brachial plexus nerve block due to the proximity of the nerves to one another.

13. B: These patients are placed in the reverse Trendelenburg position, and placement of a padded footboard helps to prevent slipping down the table and causing patient injury.

14. A: Although the preoperative and circulating RNs validate the consent form for correctness, it is the surgeon's responsibility to obtain informed consent. This is achieved by completely explaining the procedure to the patient in a manner she can understand, listing the risks, benefits, complications, and alternatives available. This conversation should also include what to expect postoperatively and which of the patient's lifestyle factors might affect the plan of care.

15. C: Although the physician that is performing the surgery should be discussed with the patient during the informed consent procedure, it is not the primary purpose. Informed consent does have a legal component and should be protected information, but its primary purpose is to inform the patient what is planned, the expected outcomes, and what are the alternatives. With the exception of emergencies, performing a procedure on a patient who has not been given proper informed consent can have legal consequences. All planned procedures should be listed on the consent form and should be addressed before the patient signs.

16. C: Surgical skin preps are meant to reduce the skin flora as much as possible by cleaning and chemically decontaminating the tissue. There is no way to sterilize or completely eliminate the skin flora. There are specific products that are used to degrease the skin, when necessary. Some surgical prep products have a degreaser product in them, but that is not the primary purpose of the prep.

17. B: Tourniquet use can cause necrosis that may require amputation later. The information recorded regarding the tourniquet includes: An assessment of the skin that will lie *under* the cuff, prior to its application; cuff location; type of material used under the cuff for skin protection; cuff pressure; calibration; time of inflation and deflation; identification, serial number and model of equipment used; name of the person applying the cuff; and an assessment of the entire extremity after use of the tourniquet.

18. B: Although all are personal safety equipment, eyewear should be specific for the laser used because the eye can absorb the laser beams. The use of a tight-fitting laser mask, not simply a surgical mask, would be appropriate.

19. D: Using a coworker's password to access EHRs, even if the record is of a patient to whom the nurse is assigned, is a violation of HIPAA. This is an intentional breach because the nurse should be aware that this is not allowed, although there is no apparent malicious intent. Additionally, doing so puts the coworker at jeopardy because an audit trail may indicate that the coworker accessed the record without authorization. If a nurse forgets a personal password, he or she should immediately contact information services to obtain a new password.

20. D: Oral intake is not given in the Phase I area, so the return of the gag reflex is not normally tested in this area, but it is in Phase II. From this area, patients are usually discharged home or to some other off-site care facility, and it is essential that the patient can tolerate fluids, if she did preoperatively.

21. B: Any facility that procures and/or stores human tissue must register with the FDA as a tissue bank. If the facility just purchases tissue for use in that facility or stores tissue for use on the same patient, this is not necessary.

22. C: The GI patient should inform the physician about any of these signs and symptoms, but the increase in abdominal swelling or pain is especially important following surgery on the liver, biliary tract, pancreas, or spleen.

23. B: There are four quadrants to the Perioperative Patient Focused Model. Three are patient focused, and one is related to the healthcare facility the care is provided.

24. C: The perioperative nurse who monitors a patient receiving local anesthetic should note the patient's skin color and condition, mental status, amount of anesthetic administered, and vital signs (BP, pulse rate and rhythm, respiration rate, and O_2 saturation). It is unnecessary to record the location of each injection.

25. B: When a perioperative nurse discovers that their perioperative patient is anxious, allay her apprehension with the proper nursing intervention: Listen attentively, provide reassurance, encourage her to express her anxiety or fear, then address it, and provide emotional support. Explaining every surgical detail would only increase her level of apprehension.

26. A: Shifting of the drapes can cause bacteria from nonprepped skin to be dragged into the sterile field. Also, the more the drape is moved, the higher the chances that it will come into contact with surrounding nonsterile furniture or fall below the sterile field.

27. C: The edges of solution containers are considered contaminated once the solutions have been poured, so they cannot be recapped for reuse, even if the cap was kept sterile.

28. C: Dorsal recumbent refers to the supine position, with the patient flat. Supine with the head of the bed lower than the feet describes the Trendelenburg position, and supine with the patient's legs elevated in stirrups is lithotomy positioning. Keeping the patient supine and elevating the entire head of the bed so it is higher than the foot is described as reverse Trendelenburg. This position would be requested in this particular surgery to provide better observation of the stomach and diaphragm.

29. A: A permanent skin marker should be used so the marking is not removed during the skin prep.

30. C: Intraoperative awareness is the rare condition in which a patient seems to be under anesthesia, but she can still hear and feel what is happening during surgery. This is affected by the depth of anesthesia, a difficult thing to monitor at times. There are now monitoring techniques such as bispectral index (BIS) monitoring that can sense the patient's brain waves through an electrode placed on the forehead. Based on the number reading, the anesthesia care provider can better determine the patient's level of consciousness.

31. B: The sterile external tie can be placed inside a sterile glove wrapper to prevent contamination when the circulator takes it to help the surgeon turn and finish tying the surgical gown.

32. A: The appropriate dosage of morphine sulfate for a pediatric patient is 0.1-0.2 mg/kg IV. MS is not well absorbed by mouth (PO) and is not recommended. Answers C and D would be too large of a dose for a pediatric patient, although the appropriate dose could be given IV, IM, or SQ.

33. B: The nurse should use the wrapper of the sterile gown to create a sterile surface away from the patient and the sterile back table. This is to prevent contamination of the sterile field by falling droplets from wet hands or inadvertently touching sterile items when picking up the gown and gloves.

34. A: The preoperative patient facing a breast biopsy experiences the fear of body image change (disfigurement), in addition to more common fears associated with surgery and anesthesia. Apprehension associated with surgical intervention and anesthesia include, but are not limited to, possible surgical outcomes, lifestyle effects, loss of control, pain, and death.

35. B: The most important piece of protective equipment used by the OR personnel during a bronchoscopy is a mask with shield and goggles. The bronchoscopy procedure causes the patient to cough uncontrollably. Washings and brushings mean tiny tissue particles will become airborne. The risk of communicable disease means the OR staff must wear masks with shields, or masks with goggles.

36. A: Ace bandages and IV tubing contain latex to make them stretchy. Symptoms of latex allergies are redness, rash, and asthmatic reactions on contact. Notify the surgeon and anesthetist immediately. Bronchitis is unlikely because the patient's History and Physical showed no respiratory disease. Since wheezing began *after* IV insertion, its most likely cause is an allergic reaction. Normal saline solution rarely causes any type of negative reaction. Fear of surgery is common, but usually presents as anxiety.

37. C: The length of time for a prep are determined by the manufacturer's recommendations and by expert studies of the effectiveness of the antimicrobial agents. Generally, these guidelines take into account the type of surgery being performed. The OR committee does not set the prep time.

38. A: In the case of multiple patients requiring simultaneous multiple procedures, the risk for wrong-site or wrong-patient errors are increased. In this scenario, factors predisposing the surgical team to make these errors include emergency surgery, unusual time pressures, multiple patients entering OR suites simultaneously, and several procedures performed on each patient.

39. C: The used surgical mask contains microorganisms from the nurse's respiratory tract and possibly from the patient. Remove the mask after surgery by handling its ties only, and then discard it into a covered container. *Never* hang a used mask around the neck, or place it in a pocket to reuse. When the mask hangs around the neck, the bacteria lose moisture and become an airborne source of contamination. Cost-savings are important, but we must not endanger the patient, visitors, or hospital personnel.

40. C: In order to continue cerebral perfusion when the carotid vessels are clamped during a carotid endarterectomy, a commercially prepared tube known as a shunt device is often used. A Javid shunt is an example of such a device.

41. B: After 30 minutes, blood products requiring refrigeration can no longer be returned to the blood bank, because the cells have already started to break down.

42. B: When a bare thumb touched the sterile glove, the glove became contaminated. Scrubbing before donning a sterile gown and gloves removes some surface bacteria, but the skin is *never* completely sterile. Discard the contaminated gloves. Ask the circulating nurse to provide a new pair. The hand is not contaminated, since what was touched was a sterile glove, but the skin contaminated the glove. There is no need to start over entirely, since only the glove is contaminated. Sterile saline cannot remove bacterial contamination from a glove.

43. C: If the nurse suspects a blood reaction, he should immediately stop the transfusion. He should then return any unused blood to the blood bank for investigation.

44. C: Although the other answers may be true, in relation to the intubation process, C is the best answer. Moving the patient before the anesthesia provider has approved may lead to accidental extubation and loss of the patient's airway, which can be life threatening.

45. B: To ensure that the sterilizers are properly sterilizing products, biological indicators should be run in them at least once a week. Implants should always have a bio run with them to ensure sterility before they are placed in a patient.

46. B: Bariatric surgery includes procedures such as gastric banding and gastric bypass, which is predominately performed for weight loss.

47. B: Shared governance is collaborative decision making between nursing personnel and hospital administration. For example, with shared governance, staff members in the surgical department may be able to set their own working schedules. However, with many staff members working 12-hour shifts, some may be resistive to adding any more tasks to their already busy schedules. The administration should begin the transition by providing education and training about the process so that the advantages are clearly outlined. Different models of shared governance include the councilor model, congress model, partnership model, collaborative model, and hybrid model.

48. C: The caffeine-halothane contracture test takes a muscle biopsy and exposes it to caffeine and halothane to check for an MH-like reaction. This test should be performed preoperatively if the patient is at risk for an MH event.

49. D: A resistive polymer blanket, which has a resistive network of wires between sheets of polymer to generate conductive warming, is a part of an active warming method. Other active heating methods include forced-air warming devices (such as the Bair Hugger), water-filled mattresses, electric blankets, carbon fiber blankets, thermal exchange chambers, negative pressure warming systems, warmed gases/fluids/irrigants, radiant warming, and warmed insufflation gases.

50. B: Normal flora are either symbiotic or commensal microorganisms that live on the patient's skin, mucous membranes, and hollow viscera. Poor aseptic technique, unclean equipment (including the overhead lights), and staff coughing, talking, and breathing may lead to infection. However, the majority of surgical site infections are traced to the patient's own normal flora becoming pathogenic.

51. A: Limiting the number of persons going in and out of the OR suite helps to lower the number of microbes allowed to enter the room. This, paired with proper air exchanges and other environmental controls, helps reduce surgical-site infections.

52. C: Draping should begin at the surgical site and move to the periphery to reduce contamination from nonprepped skin areas.

53. B: Endoscopic light sources can become very hot and may start a fire when left on surgical drapes unattended. Whenever a light is not in use, it should be placed on standby mode to prevent risk of burn injury and fire.

54. C: Nausea, vomiting, and respiratory depression are not considered therapeutic effects but rather side effects, which are not specific to midazolam hydrochloride (Versed) alone, but can occur with many medications. Although pain control can occur with the use of Versed, short-term amnesia of the pre- and intraoperative time is the medication's primary purpose for administration. Both the circulating and postanesthesia care nurse should be aware of this effect because it could be confusing for the patient, as he or she will often not even remember going into the operating suite.

55. D: Type 1 diabetic patients have a potential for dehydration, electrolyte imbalance, and inadequate circulation. These factors, among others, can cause hypertension in these patients intraoperatively. Infection and delayed wound healing are potential *postoperative* complications with diabetic patients.

56. B: It is important to document everyone present in the positioning of the patient because the patient's chart is a legal document. This information could become important should the patient sustain an injury attributed to the positioning during the surgery.

57. D: Gel has been found to be more helpful in the prevention of pressure injury formation than the traditional foam mattress. Gel is supportive to pressure points, where foam collapses. These mattresses are also less likely to crack like their foam counterparts, which can cause skin damage and create potential for infection.

58. C: Suture is sized according to gauge, similar to sewing thread. The largest gauge is #5, and the smallest is 11-0. The most commonly used sizes are #1- 4-0.

59. C: Any two licensed professionals may check the blood products before administration. This can be the circulating RN and the anesthesia care provider or two RNs. It does not need to be the nurse's patient to assist in verifying blood products.

60. D: Vicryl is the only multifilament suture listed. Multifilament sutures should not be used in infected sites because they have a characteristic referred to as capillarity, which can cause the suture to harbor bacteria and fluids.

61. C: A wedge under the patient's right side helps relieve uterine pressure off the vena cava. Laying in the other positions can risk the compression of the vena cava, which can result in both maternal and fetal decline.

62. B: A *never event* is an adverse occurrence that is plainly identifiable and measurable, results in death or major disability, and is generally preventable. *Never events* include: Surgery performed on the wrong body part or wrong patient; incorrect procedure; retention of a foreign object following surgery; medication error or contaminated drug; inappropriate equipment use; IV air embolism; incompatible blood transfusion; stage 3 or 4 pressure injuries from improper positioning; wrong inhalation agent; a burn, fall, or death of an ASA Class 1 patient.

63. B: If a patient can physically assist with transfer, a minimum of two staff members are needed to stand on either side of the bed to prevent falls. If the patient is unable to assist, then a minimum of four team members are needed.

64. C: Sutures, along with clips, clamps, and tourniquets are examples of manual hemostasis. The laser and ESU are thermal agents. Fibrin glue is a chemical hemostasis agent.

65. A: The scrub nurse should dry from the fingers upward without retracing an area. This helps to prevent contamination of the cleansed areas.

66. C: The circulating nurse should report all deaths in the OR to the coroner's office for review. This information can usually be found on the "death packet" paperwork or in the facility's policy for management of death in the operating room. No lines or drains should be removed from the patient until the coroner's office has released the patient. This is especially important for cases where criminal activity may have been involved.

67. C: Chemical indicators test the conditions within the sterilizer. These indicators do not indicate sterility, just that the parameters of the sterilization cycle have been met. Biological indicators are the only way to assure sterility, because they have living spores inside that are resistant to sterilizing agents. The biological indicators are tested after the cycle, and if the contained spores are dead, it proves that the item is truly sterile.

68. C: Sorbitol is routinely used as a urologic irrigation that is an integral part of a cystoscopy.

69. D: The minimum recommended distance is 12 inches or 1 foot. Although 15 inches is technically a correct option, it is not the minimum distance asked for in the question. This distance is the agreed-upon "safe" distance by perioperative professional organizations so as to prevent inadvertent contamination.

70. A: When the surgeon gives a verbal order for medication during surgery, written confirmation of the drug and dosage is the preferred method for *verifying* the order. The surgeon, not the scrub nurse, is the person who substantiates medication and dosage. The perioperative nurse must check the patient's record for allergies prior to administering any medication, but this is not part of the verification process. A newly ordered medication during the surgery is not entered in the patient's record until the surgeon updates it, following the procedure.

71. B: Although this information should be verified with the patient in the preoperative area, the final "time out" should be immediately before the procedure starts, after draping, and it should be repeated for each additional procedure. It is important to be sure that any surgical site marks are visible after draping so they may be verified in the time-out process.

72. B: To prevent the risk of needle sticks, sharps are always placed in a puncture-proof container specifically designed for them, not any type of trash bag. Because the sharps discussed in this question cannot be reprocessed, the nurse would not put them in a container to be resterilized.

73. B: Lasers of any kind can be a safety hazard and should always be placed in "standby" mode when not in use. Usually, the equipment tech will do this automatically, but the surgical team members should also be aware to avoid injury.

74. A: Holding the drapes above the OR table prevents the edges from being contaminated. Draping should start from the site and proceed outward, because the site is sterile and the other areas are not.

75. A: Nonsterile equipment is sometimes needed for a procedure. If it can be sterilized, then the nurse should do so. If not, the best option is to cover it with a sterile drape to prevent contamination to the sterile field. Many vendors make drapes for specific items used in surgery that cannot be sterilized, such as C-arm drapes.

76. A: The Joint Commission instituted a standardized approach to "hand-off" communications between perioperative personnel. The Holding Area nurse must provide *appropriate* information to the perioperative circulating nurse, which includes discussion of the proper surgical site, but is not limited to it.

77. C: Because the recipient site is considered contaminated in this case; it should be prepped last to prevent inadvertent contamination of the donor site. It is recommended to use a colorless prep, so the surgeon can evaluate the vascular supply to the donor skin. If there is not proper vascularity, the donor skin will not survive on the recipient site.

78. D: The nurse should always start counting items on the surgical field, and then the back table, followed by the items that have been passed off the surgical field, also referred to as the floor count. Counting in a consistent manner, starting at the surgical field will help prevent delays in wound closure and miscounts.

79. D: The ASA physical status classification system has six classes. Healthy patients are ASA I. ASA II is mild disease, III is severe, IV is life threatening, and V applies to patients that are not expected to live more than 24 hours. Brain death would be considered ASA VI.

80. D: Because the effects of any regional anesthesia should be worn off by the time the patient reaches Phase II, motor and sensory function are not a normal assessment area.

81. B: The perioperative nurse must understand anatomy, surgical procedures, instruments, OR equipment, and perioperative safety among other areas of expertise. The anesthesiologist or nurse anesthetist performs endotracheal tube insertion. The perioperative nurse assists with intubation, but is not responsible for identifying internal physical landmarks to ensure tube placement is correct.

82. B: The circulating perioperative nurse relays updates from the surgeon to the patient's family via telephone to the Waiting Room. (Often, a hospital volunteer screens the call to ensure the nurse is speaking with the correct person.) The first obligation is to the patient, but the circulating nurse should also keep the family informed. Leaving the OR to go to the Waiting Room is unnecessary.

83. C: Without proper padding and extremity placement, the lateral position can cause nerve damage to the extremities, such as the brachial plexus. Lower back strain could occur with lithotomy. Pressure injuries to the back of the head would be more consistent with a supine position or some version of it. Skin tears on the buttocks result from shearing forces. These types of injuries are a risk of the reverse Trendelenburg position.

84. D: The Meals on Wheels program provides low-cost meals to patients who are homebound. Most programs have a sliding scale for people with limited income, and some programs accept donations in place of a set fee, but overall costs are often no more or even less than buying groceries. Most programs include a hot meal at lunchtime, a sandwich or small meal for evening, and cereal and fruit for breakfast. Meals are designed to meet the nutritional needs of older adults, and specialized diets (such as low sodium) are often available.

85. D: Sponge counts should be done before the case, at the closure of each cavity, before the wound is closed, after the wound is closed, and upon any permanent relief of staff.

86. C: There are three types of dermatomes, and they are used for removing tissue that will be used in skin grafting.

87. C: University of Wisconsin (UW) solution, or ViaSpan, is a medication used as an organ flush after harvesting in preparation for transplant. Of the choices listed, a living donor nephrectomy would be the only correct choice.

88. A: Smoking causes vasoconstriction and thereby compromises blood flow to the periphery of the body and puts the tissues at risk. This places these patients at a higher risk for pressure injury or ulcer formation.

89. D: The nurse would give 2.5 mg/kg IV initially and repeat dosing until signs and symptoms abate, up to 10 mg/kg. The nurse may need to increase the concentration to stop the signs and symptoms from continuing.

90. A: Dantrolene sodium (Dantrium) is a skeletal muscle relaxant. Dantrium is the drug of choice for treating the rigid muscles and fever associated with malignant hyperthermia. If a patient experiences malignant hyperthermia, the anesthetist should discontinue the triggering anesthetic (usually halothane). Hyperventilate the patient with 100% O_2. Administer Dantrium by rapid IV push, 1 mg/kg. Do not mix Dantrium with D5W or normal saline. The doctor may order more Dantrium at three-minute intervals, for a total of 10 mg/kg, and add bromocriptine. If possible, terminate the surgery.

91. B: Because of the need of thoracic cross clamping during these surgeries, the spinal cord may become ischemic from the lack of blood flow. This is especially true if the cross-clamping lasts longer than 30 minutes. The patient's risk of stroke or previous spine surgery would be an additional patient-specific risk factor, not one associated with the procedure itself.

92. C: In the Kraske position, the patient is placed prone and the foot of the bed is lowered. Then the entire bed is tilted so the patient's hips are higher than the rest of the body. This position greatly increases visualization in rectal surgery cases. A total vaginal hysterectomy would be in the lithotomy position. A total abdominal hysterectomy and a thyroidectomy would be in the supine position.

93. C: Bupivacaine, or Marcaine, is a common local anesthetic medication used in epidural anesthesia. Meperidine is a narcotic. Bacitracin is an antibiotic, and succinylcholine is a paralytic agent used as a muscle relaxant in general anesthesia.

94. A: Personnel who must remain close to the surgical field, such as the scrubbed team members, should wear thyroid shields and leaded glasses because these areas are very sensitive to radiation exposure.

95. B: Only the top of a sterilely draped back table is actually considered sterile, not the edges or sides. Any sterile item that extends past the edge of the sterile area is no longer considered sterile and should be discarded immediately. Although the sterile scrub tech would not want to touch the contaminated tip, she can discard it by touching the part still on the table or remove it from the field so the circulator can discard it. A nonsterile person should never reach over or onto a sterile field to retrieve an item.

96. B: Chemical manufacturers provide a safety data sheet (SDS, formerly MSDS) for each chemical they sell. The SDS describes the dangers of each chemical and first-aid measures in the event of exposure. If the SDS cannot be found, the Safety Officer should be called.

97. C: A double-cuff tourniquet is used for this procedure. In a Bier block, once the tourniquet is placed, the patient's arm is elevated and wrapped with a compression bandage (Esmarch) to remove blood from the distal portion of the extremity. The upper cuff of the tourniquet is then inflated. The local medication is injected through an intravenous line in that extremity. Once the medication has anesthetized the extremity, the lower cuff of the tourniquet is inflated, and the upper cuff is released.

98. C: To prevent injury, sharps should be passed in a "hands-free" manner in a safe zone, such as placing the knife handle in an emesis basin.

99. D: Elderly patients may have more drug interactions because their tolerance and detoxification through the kidneys and liver are often lower than in their younger counterparts. Because this population often has lower body fat as well, fat-soluble medications, such as many anesthetic agents, may metabolize slower and cause a dangerous interaction with pain control medications.

100. B: Loupes are magnifying eyeglasses that the surgeon wears during microsurgery, in this case to see the small sutures used in the procedure.

101. A: The general recommendation for hair at the surgical site is to leave it in place. Shaving increases the risk of postoperative infection, and little advantage has been shown from hair removal, although hair may at times be removed if it obscures vision of the surgical field, interferes with closure of the wound, prevents drapes or dressings from adhering, or creates a fire risk. If removal is indicated, the minimal amount necessary should be removed as near to the time of surgery as possible.

102. A: The safety strap helps secure the patient, preventing falls, and it should be placed across her thighs. A strap across the chest could impede respirations and is not as secure. Due to the narrow width of most OR tables, a safety strap should be placed whether the patient is sedated or not, even if other staff is available to secure her. Should the patient move unexpectedly, she could still fall and injury herself and the staff members who try to catch her.

103. B: Class 2 therapeutic compression stockings, which are commonly used as VTE prophylaxis after surgery, provide pressure of 30–40 mmHg. The stockings come in many sizes and colors and may extend from the foot to the knee or the groin. The stockings must be fitted properly and must have the correct level of compression:

- Class 1: 20–30 mmHg (varicose veins)
- Class 2: 30–40 mmHg (venous ulcers and prophylaxis)
- Class 3: 40–50 mmHg (refractory venous ulcers and lymphedema)
- Class 4: 50–60 mmHg (lymphedema)

104. B: Allogenous refers to blood that is collected from a donor other than oneself. Blood substitutes are oxygen-carrying products that are alternatives to giving actual blood, whereas blood volume expanders only add volume and have no oxygen-carrying component. Autologous blood transfusions, or autotransfusion, refers to collecting a patient's own blood and returning it to them. This can be achieved through a preoperative donation or intraoperatively with the use of a blood salvage unit.

105. A: Supination, or palms facing up, when the arms are extended helps to prevent ulnar nerve damage in the supine position. All other answers could result in injury.

106. C: The optimal score with the Aldrete postanesthesia scoring system is a 10. There are five areas that are assessed; each is scored 0-2 points. Although this patient is fully awake, moving, and back to preanesthetic circulatory function, she is not breathing deeply and still needs oxygen to keep her saturation above 92. These last two areas would be scored as a 1 instead of the optimal 2, giving the patient an Aldrete score of 8.

107. A: Even though the 1–10 numeric scale for describing pain is ubiquitous in health care in the United States, it is not commonly used in many other cultures, such as the Mexican culture, so it can be confusing to patients, who may be unsure how to respond. The most appropriate intervention is to ask the patient to describe the pain in a different way, such as mild (*leve*), moderate (*moderado*), or severe (*severo*). If the patient speaks minimal or no English, an interpreter may be needed to ascertain the patient's level of pain.

108. A: Chlorhexidine gluconate is the only antiseptic solution on this list that is an ingredient in many surgical preps. Acetone is used as an effective degreaser, but by itself it does not have antiseptic qualities. ChloraPrep is actually a skin prep product that is made up of chlorhexidine gluconate and alcohol.

109. C: According to current National Patient Safety Goals and the Surgical Care Improvement Project (SCIP), antibiotics should be administered within 1 hour of incision for best practice effectiveness.

110. A: Warning signs should be placed so anyone entering the room will know that the laser is in use. Although the nurse should not store liquids on the laser equipment, the scrub tech should have a bowl of sterile water or saline solution available in case of a fire. When the laser is not in use, it should be kept in "standby," even if the surgeon requests it to remain armed. This is to prevent inadvertent firing that could injure the patient or team. Finally, a halon extinguisher, not an ABC-type extinguisher should be available.

111. A: The BIS monitor has a range in readings from 100 to 0. A 100 reading on the BIS monitor means the patient is fully awake, and 0 is no brain activity.

112. C: To prevent hypothermia, IV fluids are typically warmed to a maximum temperature of 106 °F (41 °C). If heated in a warming cabinet, the IV fluids will begin to cool fairly rapidly after being removed. Warmed IV fluids are usually used as an adjunct to other warming methods, such as warmed anesthesia gases, active or passive heating of the body, warmed insufflation gases, and warmed irrigating solutions.

113. C: ESWL, also known as extracorporeal shock wave lithotripsy, is a procedure that uses shock waves to break up kidney stones so the patient may excrete them safely.

114. C: A Litvak Pereyra needle is a ligature needle used in bladder neck suspensions to help pull the sutures of the suspension mesh upward and secure them.

115. B: Benchmarking and interventions are elements of the AORN Perioperative Patient Focused Model. Communicating is a human response pattern discussed by North American Nursing Diagnosis Association (NANDA). Planning is the only answer that is a step in the nursing process. Planning is needed to create the necessary interventions for the surgical patient, her problem, and potential problems. It is during this phase that caregivers should include the patient's input in their plan of care.

116. A: Surgical specimens should be specially handled and listed as either surgical pathology examination (routine), gross examination, or disposal. Frozen section and permanent are examples of surgical pathology.

117. C: The internal ties are the only ones that are not in contact with the exterior sterile portion of the gown; therefore, they are the only ones the circulator or other nonsterile team members may touch to help gown the surgeon.

118. D: The operating room department is made up of three areas: unrestricted, semirestricted, and restricted. In the unrestricted areas, such as the front office, surgical personnel can wear street clothes. In semirestricted areas, which usually refer to areas inside the department but not inside the suite, surgical personnel need to wear authorized scrub attire and hair covering. A mask is not required in these areas. The restricted areas include anywhere that sterile supplies are opened, such as the actual OR suite. In these areas, proper attire and a mask must be worn.

119. A: The draping materials form a barrier and must be fluid resistant and resistant to tearing or puncture to avoid microbial penetration. A sterile drape should be lint free to reduce airborne contaminates and shedding onto the surgical site.

120. C: By pulling up the sleeves of the gown, it allows the surgeon's fingers and hand to pass into the awaiting sterile glove easier. The other answers may cause the scrub nurse to contaminate her sterile gloves.

121. B: Bacterial spores are the most resistant due to their capacity to withstand external destructive agents.

122. C: Jackknife positioning is another name for the Kraske position.

123. B: Ethylene oxide, EO, is the only type of chemical agent listed. Steam is a form of thermal agent. Microwave and X ray are forms of radiation agents.

124. D: Freedom from infection is an extremely important desired outcome. Excellent aseptic technique, including the proper prepping of the incision site and proper draping methods, contributes to the desired outcome of freedom from infection. The anesthetic agent itself does not have a major effect on the incidence of infection.

125. A: The three modes of transmission for microorganisms in the OR are droplet, airborne and contact. Body fluids, purulent material, blood, sneezing, coughing, talking, and dirty equipment are possible sources of contamination, which are included under the three modes of transmission.

126. D: Plavix is usually stopped within 48 hours of cardiac surgery. Warfarin, also known as Coumadin, should be stopped 5 to 7 days prior to surgery. Diuretics, such as Lasix, should be stopped the morning of surgery, but it is usually not necessary to stop aspirin prior to this surgery.

127. C: Hypokalemia is characterized by premature ventricular contractions (PVCs) because adequate potassium levels are needed to maintain cardiac electrical stability. Additionally, hypokalemia can result in increased excitability of ventricular cells, so they are more likely to have premature contractions. With PVCs, an electrocardiogram (ECG) reading shows wide distorted QRS complexes. Hypoxemia can also result in PVCs, so oxygen saturation should be carefully monitored. Treatment for hypokalemia is potassium supplementation.

128. A: If a pneumatic tourniquet is used for more than 75 minutes on a pediatric patient, the patient should be assessed with arterial blood gases for acidosis because products of anaerobic metabolism enter the systemic circulation when the cuff is released. One study, for example, showed that lactic acid was elevated for 10 minutes after removal of the pneumatic cuff. Generally, authorities recommend that the use of pneumatic tourniquets be limited to 75 minutes for pediatric patients for this reason.

129. B: In order to avoid confusion, it is recommended that the surgeon write YES or their initials on the surgical site. Other methods can be confusing and lead to a wrong-site surgery.

130. B: Carbon dioxide is used to insufflate the abdomen during laparoscopic cases. The other gases listed would be toxic to the patient if used in this manner.

131. B: Postmortem identification tags are specific to identification of deceased patients. One should be placed on the patient, usually on the toe, and another on the outside of the shroud.

132. D: All the other items are detectable on a radiograph except nonradiopaque towels. For this reason, they should never be used in a wound due to the risk of retention.

133. C: As long as the fluid is not expired, the nurse can keep it after it is removed from the warming cabinet but cannot rewarm it. It is recommended that the nurse places a "Do Not Rewarm" label on the bottle and store it at room temperature until the manufacturer's recommended expiration date.

134. B: A person with a body mass index of 40 or above, or 35 to 40 with serious comorbidities would be a potential candidate for bariatric surgery.

135. A: Of the four choices, only an ESU uses electrical current to manipulate the patient's tissues. In order to complete the electrical circuit and not harm the patient, electricity flows from the unit (generator) to the active electrode (Bovie pencil) and is returned to the generator by the return patient electrode, also known as the inactive dispersive electrode, rather than through the patient or team members.

136. C: Roux-en-Y gastric bypass is the only procedure listed that is a combination of the two bariatric surgery approaches: restrictive and malabsorptive. Both proximal gastric bypass and banding are restrictive, and jejunoileal bypass is a malabsorptive.

137. A: Frequent monitoring of vital signs will help the PACU nurse identify any complications in a timely manner. Each hospital may have a policy regarding vital sign monitoring, such as every 5 minutes for the first 20 minutes, then every 15 minutes throughout the postoperative stay. Others may require vitals every 5 minutes throughout the entire first hour.

138. C: The magnetic field of an MRI scan is considered safe for the general public beyond the 5 gauss line. The magnetic field of the earth is approximately 0.5 gauss. A 1 Tesla MRI is equal to 10,000 gauss. Electronic devices and ferromagnetic objects cannot be brought inside the 5 gauss line. Ferrous metal objects may become projectiles if exposed to the high magnetic fields of the MRI machine, and implanted metal prostheses or other devices may rotate.

139. A: When a patient is placed prone, or on her stomach, chest rolls are used to help relieve the weight on the chest. This allows for better lung expansion and adequate breathing. Stirrups are used for lithotomy positions. Footboards are useful in reverse Trendelenburg positioning, and beanbags are mostly used in lateral positions.

140. B: Keeping the doors closed helps to reduce the number of microbes in the OR suite. This is true whether a surgery is occurring or not.

141. D: In this situation, only the radiology tech should be moving the C-arm. Only trained personnel with proper state licensing should operate these devices.

142. C: Only areas from the chest to the sterile field, and two inches above the elbow and gloves are sterile. The back of the gown and below the waist are not considered sterile.

143. A: The read-back procedure when taking a verbal or telephone order is used primarily to ensure the accuracy of the order. If there is a series of orders, the nurse should read back the orders after each order is given rather than performing a read back of all orders at the end. Each item should be read back in totality, exactly as given; any questions about the order, such as clarification of a dosage, should be asked at that time and repeated back as well.

144. D: All of the above items should be removed before surgery, but only the nail polish/acrylic nail choice can interfere with the anesthesia monitoring of the patient. Many pulse oximeters, used for oxygen saturation monitoring, are placed on the finger and require visualization of the nail bed to properly function. Nail bed color is also used as an indicator of peripheral circulation. The patient should be instructed that if she wears these items, she should uncover at least one fingernail.

145. B: Rigid containers weigh up to 10 pounds. Condensation may occur on the surfaces of a rigid container, contaminating the entire package (referred to as "wet pack"). Despite these drawbacks, rigid packaging is durable and provides excellent defense against damage to the contents.

146. C: It is recommended that surgical attire be low linting to prevent foreign bodies' entrance into the sterile area. It should be changed daily, even if it has not become soiled. Although disposable scrubs are acceptable, reusable ones can also be used as long as they meet the proper requirements.

147. B: CO_2 gas is inserted into an abdominal cavity either through a percutaneous method using a Veress needle or by the open technique using a trocar.

148. A: Chromic gut is the only suture from the list that is both a monofilament and an absorbable suture. Nylon and polypropylene (Prolene) are nonabsorbable. Vicryl, although absorbable, is a multifilament suture.

149. A: The circulating nurse documents the type and amount of irrigation, fluid output, and blood products. The circulating nurse does *not* record the amount of prep solution used.

150. C: Just because a patient has cochlear implants, it does not mean that the patient is adept at understanding spoken language, especially if he or she received the cochlear implants as an adult and had a long history of deafness. The brain needs time to properly interpret sounds, and people develop varying degrees of successful hearing, so the nurse should ask if the patient needs a sign language interpreter or would like to use another means of communication. If the patient has a good ability to interpret sounds, the nurse should face the patient and speak slowly and clearly to aid comprehension.

151. A: Although reference labs may vary slightly, generally, a total bilirubin level greater than 13 mg/dL is considered a critical value for a newborn; for adults and children, a critical value is a level greater than 15 mg/dL. The normal total bilirubin level for a neonate (day 1) is less than 5.8 mg/dL. Bilirubin is a by-product of heme catabolism and is produced primarily in the liver, spleen, and bone marrow. Increased bilirubin may be the result of prehepatic, hepatic, or posthepatic conditions. As bilirubin levels increase, yellow pigment is deposited in the skin and sclera, resulting in jaundice.

152. A: Assess the patient's skin both prior to and after surgery. Note the type of equipment used for positioning, such as stirrups for lithotomy position, placement of the extremities, and special precautions used to protect the eyes. Record any changes in the patient's position, the location of the safety strap, and the name of the person who positioned the patient. The height of the operating table and Mayo stand, and the number of staff assisting the surgeon do not affect the patient's position. If the table is elevated during the procedure, check the Mayo stand to ensure it does not rest directly on the patient.

153. C: Atrial fibrillation is the most common cardiac arrhythmia following aortic valve replacement surgery, at a rate of approximately 12% according to the American College of Cardiology. Atrial fibrillation can have an acute or late onset and increases risk for stroke and mortality for those individuals.

154. D: Although some bleeding into the tissues along the incision may occur during a surgical procedure, if the area is firm, erythematous, and raised, this likely suggests a hematoma, which is an accumulation of blood in the tissues. The raised area may be evident before the discoloration appears, depending on the depth. Small hematomas often resolve without intervention, but their size and location should be carefully reported and documented because bleeding can become severe. Ecchymoses may look similar, but they are flat rather than raised.

155. A: Although the temperature may be adjusted for patient safety, 68-73 °F is the recommended temperature range to keep the patient normothermic. Warmer temperatures may increase the growth of harmful organisms in the surgical suite. In addition, humidity may be affected by temperature changes outside this optimal range. Increases in humidity can also harbor microorganism growth.

156. C: Shellfish allergy can indicate an allergy to iodine. Many contrast media contain iodine. Contrast is a necessary component in endovascular procedures due to the use of x ray. This would not affect antibiotic choice or be indicative of a latex allergy. An allergy to eggs might affect the use of propofol.

157. A: Meperidine (12.5–25 mg IV) is commonly used to control the severe shivering associated with hypothermia, although shivering may also occur in normothermic patients, especially after general anesthesia. Shivering is uncomfortable and may increase operative pain. Additionally, shivering increases oxygen consumption by up to 400%, which can result in hypoxemia. Females tend to experience episodes of postoperative shivering more often than do males. Generally, nonpharmacologic interventions, such as forced-air heating blankets and warmed IV fluids, are used before medications are tried. Other medications used to control shivering include tramadol, clonidine, low-dose ketamine, and dexmedetomidine.

158. C: Risk increases the longer the surgery is, but studies show it dramatically increases after three hours. If possible, efforts should be made to reposition the patient after this time. If this is not possible, careful inspection and documentation of the skin integrity should take place when the surgery ends.

159. B: During a decortication of a lung, the restrictive tissue is stripped away from the pleura to enhance respiration.

160. B: The nurse should open the door and leave the items inside to dry. Fifteen to sixty minutes is the recommended drying time for steam sterilizers, but this range varies by manufacturer. The nurse would not want to remove the items and put them away or leave them on a table because the items will still be very warm. Placing them on a cold surface could cause condensation on the surface and put the items at risk for contamination from strike-through of the collected fluid. There is no separate "dry" cycle for these sterilizers.

161. A: It is impossible to clear the skin entirely of microorganisms and spores. Even a strong antiseptic solution, such as povidone iodine, cannot make skin completely sterile, but just reduces the number of microorganisms. The purpose of aseptic practice is to prevent the invasion of microorganisms into the open incision, and to create and maintain the integrity of a sterile field surrounding the wound, isolating it from the merely clean adjacent areas.

162. C: Ketamine is the only answer that is both given intravenously and is a general anesthetic agent that is commonly administered to children. It is a short-acting and effective sedative with neuro-protective qualities that also preserves both cardiac and respiratory function.

163. B: There are five variations of these three categories: conventional cutting, reverse cutting, side cutting, tapered, and blunt.

164. A: Many sharps, such as hypodermic needles and suture needles, are not recommended for reprocessing. In addition, suture material itself can have decreased strength if reprocessed. Trocars, endoscopic graspers and opened and unused sutures are commonly reprocessed.

165. D: Dantrolene use has reduced the mortality associated with an MH crisis from 70% to less than 10% and while this reaction is rare, it's a critical medication in the OR environment. Propofol is an anesthetic agent. Succinylcholine is a muscle relaxant used in the induction of anesthesia. Lasix is a diuretic and least relevant in the operating room.

166. B: When a unidirectional ultraclean air delivery system is in use, the surgical site and the instrument tables should be within the air curtain. The air curtain is the area in which clean air flows constantly, creating essentially a room within a room. Obstacles to the air flow (including lights, microscopes, team members) can decrease the effectiveness of the air flow. With a system that uses a horizontal air flow, it is important to avoid standing between the air curtain and the surgical site or instrument tables.

167. C: The five rights of safe medication administration include right patient, drug, dose, route and time. The missing component is right time. The right time is verified by checking the physician order for the administration time or, in the case of PRN medications, checking how frequently the medication can be provided and when the last dose was administered.

168. C: Sudden revascularization of the operative limb in fem-pop bypass patients may lead to operative leg swelling. Although the other answers are possible complications, they are very rare.

169. C: *Exogenous* sources of infection come from outside the body, including the environment and hospital personnel, such as cracks in nail polish, artificial nails, jewelry, talking/coughing/breathing, or the use of contaminated surgical instruments and supplies. The patient's skin flora provides an *endogenous* source of infection because it comes from inside the body and it is always present.

170. A: A special consideration for correct draping is to ensure that the prep solutions have dried before applying surgical drapes. Pooled prep fluids can cause skin breakdown. These fluids, especially those containing alcohol, can also be flammable when still in liquid form.

171. C: Although keeping track of fluids in and out will help with the determination of blood loss, the most important reason is to determine if a fluid deficit is occurring. In this particular surgery, the patient can absorb fluid media into the vascular system, which can cause many complications, and even death.

172. A: The CO_2 gas insufflated into the abdomen causes a space to be formed in the cavity, so the surgeon can better visualize the internal structures and have space to work.

173. B: Symptoms of MH can reoccur for up to 72 hours after an incident and initial dantrolene administration, therefore the Malignant Hypothermia Association of the US recommends that IV dantrolene (in boluses or continuous infusion) be continued for at least 24 hours after the incident occurred, after which the dose can be titrated down based on patient status.

174. C: The main differences between these two types of OR suite cleaning is that turnover cleaning is done between each surgery, and terminal cleaning is done at the end of the day and is a more complete cleaning.

175. C: Beck's triad is an indicator of an acute cardiac tamponade.

176. A: Wrapping materials used during the sterilization process must meet certain safety standards, such as resistance to tears, punctures, and abrasions. Other requirements include: Enough porosity to allow for steam or gas penetration and venting; effective air and microorganism barrier; secure enclosure of contents; moisture resistance (*not water-proof*); absence of toxic ingredients and non-fast dyes; sufficient seal integrity; aseptic delivery of contents to the sterile field; correct labeling; adequate size for even content distribution; and ability to sustain the sterility of contents until opening.

177. B: The insufflated CO_2 gas is measured in mmHg, and although the intra-abdominal pressure may be adjusted by the surgeon to better meet the needs of the patient, the recommended level is 12-15 mmHg.

178. B: The scrub nurse carefully picks up the towel by a corner, with one hand. This is to prevent water from dropping on the towel and contaminating it.

179. A: It is important for a "time out" to be called before any procedure, including regional anesthetic procedures. The patient should have been identified at the preoperative level and with the anesthesia care provider when first brought into the OR suite.

180. D: It is very important to carefully handle and document forensic specimens from the time of removal from the patient to examination. This information establishes the chain of custody of this evidence. This is particularly important if the specimen is involved in a criminal investigation.

181. B: The patient is screened and prepared for an intraoperative magnetic resonance imaging (MRI) scan in MRI zone II. Zones are as follows:

- Zone I: General public area that is typically a waiting area.
- Zone II: Preparation area where the patient is screened in preparation for the MRI scan. Access is through controlled access doors.

- Zone III: Caution zone—access is restricted to screened MRI patients and personnel only.
- Zone IV: Danger zone (the scanner room), access is restricted to screened MRI patients under direct supervision of MRI personnel.

182. A: The most commonly used preservative for biological specimens is 10% formalin, which is a solution of formaldehyde. The specimen should be fully immersed in the preservative, and the lowest ratio of formalin volume that will provide effective preservation should be used. Formaldehyde is carcinogenic, so alternatives to formalin are under research, but no recommendations have as yet been made. Vacuum-based preservation is one alternative currently under consideration.

183. D: The United Network of Organ Sharing (UNOS) identifies each organ for transplant with a special number known as the UNOS number.

184. C: Although the surgeon might suggest it, the nurse should never warm irrigation or IV fluids by placing them in the microwave or a warm autoclave. Because there is no temperature control with these methods, the patient and team members could sustain burn injuries with this method. The most effective way to safely heat fluids is through the use of a specially designed fluid warming cabinet or a portable fluid warmer. These items are set at the recommended range and have a digital readout so the nurse may verify the safe temperature of the fluids before use on the patient.

185. B: This age group tends to experience separation anxiety when separated from parents. Body image concerns are more appropriate in the teen years. Four to six year olds may act like fantasy characters when confronted with stressful situations, and nonverbal sounds would be more appropriate for infant-age patients.

186. C: Any surgery where the team sees a risk for a retained instrument, instrument counts should be performed. These counts are done at the same frequency as sponge and sharp counts.

187. C: The blood urea nitrogen level is used to assess kidney function. The liver produces urea and nitrogen as waste products, which are then filtered through the kidneys. If the kidneys are not functioning properly, these waste products increase in the blood.

Age	Normal Value	Critical Value (nondialysis patients)
0-3	5–17 mg/dL	>40 mg/dL
4-13	7–17 mg/dL	>55 mg/dL
14-adult	8–21 mg/dL	>100 mg/dL
>90	10–31 mg/dL	>100 mg/dL

188. C: A Maryland dissector forceps is an endoscopic instrument most commonly used in laparoscopic procedures. In this case, the laparoscopic cholecystectomy is the only option in which this instrument would be used.

189. B: Spinal cord injury is the only listed complication of a thoracotomy that is not also shared by VAT surgery.

190. D: Dextran is a nonelectrolyte fluid that is safe with monopolar electrosurgery, but it is a derivative of beet sugar and should not be used on persons with this allergy, allergy to the fluid media itself, or hemostatic illnesses. It is not recommended to use more than 500 mL of this solution during the surgery.

191. B: Wearing surgical attire helps prevent bacterial shedding from the human body, in the form of hair, dead skin, and other particles. It also helps control the surgical environment by eliminating items from outside that might be on a perioperative personnel's clothing that could cause a surgical site infection, such as pet hair.

192. A: Compressed air and nitrogen are the only two gas sources that should be used with a pneumatic tourniquet. Nitrous oxide and oxygen should never be used because they increase the risk of fire.

193. A: Although it could happen to any of these instruments, the nurse shouldn't place a needle holder on an instrument magnet because it could become magnetized. Because the purpose of this instrument is to safely manipulate suture needles, if the instrument becomes magnetized it may not properly release the needle or attract it back and cause injury to the sterile team or the patient.

194. B: Sterile packages require pressure-sensitive chemical indicator tape that is specific to the type of sterilization technique (steam, dry heat, or gas). Black stripes appear on the autoclave tape when the pack is correctly sterilized. Surgical adhesive, paper tape, and water-resistant tape are inappropriate for use on a sterile package.

195. C: Nerve, epidural, and intrathecal blocks, which tend to be used during a carpal tunnel release, are all forms of regional anesthesia.

196. A: Supplies without a posted expiration date are considered sterile until the package is opened or integrity is compromised. This is called "event-related" sterility.

197. A: The medications given to the patient for general anesthesia can be very disorienting and frightening for the patient. It is important for the circulating nurse to stay at the bedside to comfort the patient and to assist the anesthesia provider as needed in case there is a complication.

198. D: Per JCAHO recommendations, the person with the most knowledge of the patient and planned procedure should mark the patient. This is usually the surgeon.

199. C: The perioperative nurse performs a variety of functions, including patient assessment, development of a nursing diagnosis, and implementation of the plan of care. During the perioperative phase, the nurse assembles pertinent patient information, identifies desired outcomes, then develops and executes a plan of care. Generally, the primary care provider creates the discharge plan, and because the patient is never discharged directly from the OR, the perioperative nurse is not involved in the implementation of that plan.

200. D: The circulating nurse is responsible for transporting the patient to the OR, taking report from the Holding Area nurse, and relaying patient information to the other perioperative staff. Passing instruments to the surgeon during surgery is the responsibility of the scrub nurse.

It's Your Moment, Let's Celebrate It!

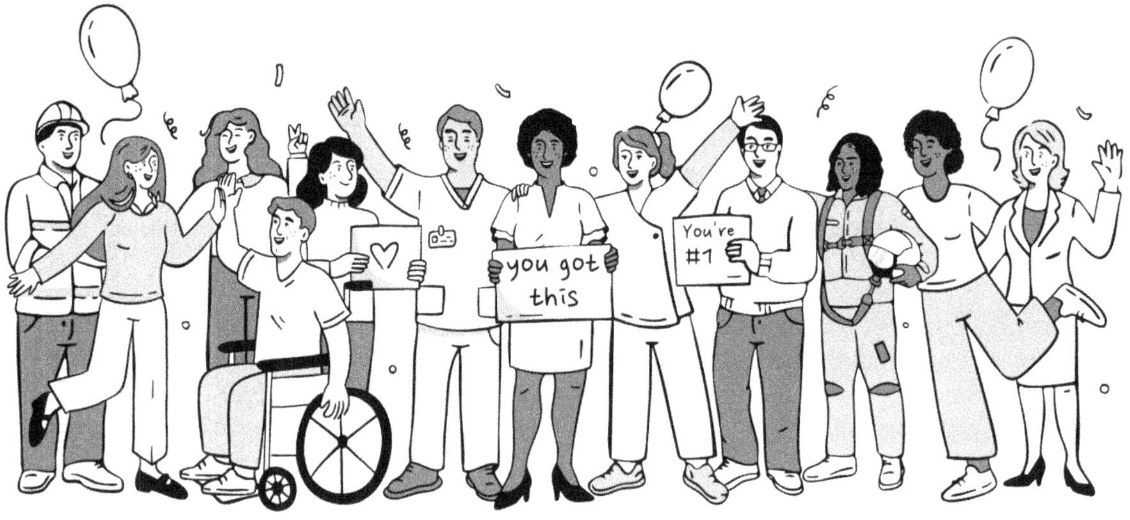

Share your story @mometrixtestpreparation

www.ingramcontent.com/pod-product-compliance
Lightning Source LLC
Chambersburg PA
CBHW061327190326
41458CB00011B/3917
* 9 7 8 1 5 1 6 7 0 7 9 5 9 *